Human Physiology: Age, Stress, and the Environment

Second Edition

Editors

R.M. CASE

and J.M. WATERHOUSE

Oxford   New York   Tokyo

OXFORD UNIVERSITY PRESS

Oxford University Press, Walton Street, Oxford OX2 6DP
Oxford New York
Athens Auckland Bangkok Bombay
Calcutta Cape Town Dar es Salaam Delhi
Florence Hong Kong Istanbul Karachi
Kuala Lumpur Madras Madrid Melbourne
Mexico City Nairobi Paris Singapore
Taipei Tokyo Toronto
and associated companies in
Berlin Ibadan

Oxford is a trade mark of Oxford University Press

Published in the United States by
Oxford University Press Inc., New York

© Oxford University Press, 1994

First edition published by Manchester University Press, 1985
Second edition published by Oxford University Press, 1994
Reprinted 1995

A catalogue record for this book is available from the British Library

Library of Congress Cataloging in Publication Data available

ISBN 0 19 262265 X (Hbk)
ISBN 0 19 262264 1 (Pbk)

Printed in Great Britain by
Bookcraft (Bath) Ltd, Midsomer Norton, Avon

PREFACE

Textbooks of physiology tend to focus largely on 'standard' physiology, that is, the physiology of young, 70 kg men. In reality, of course, the majority of the population do not fit this norm and this book focuses on such 'non-standard' physiology. Firstly, it describes the variations which occur in human physiology at different stages of life. Secondly, it explores the physiological responses evoked by various challenging environments, by exercise, and by trauma. In summary, it seeks to reach those parts of physiology other textbooks seldom reach.

The book is written for those who have a basic knowledge of 'standard' physiology acquired, for example, during the early stages of a course in medicine, or dentistry, or a science course in physiology.

The aim has been to apply this basic knowledge to explain the responses of the body to changed circumstances. Each of these circumstances is explored in a separate chapter and, though there is a natural progression of subject matter, each chapter stands alone and can be read in isolation.

This book has two main messages. Firstly, that there is no such thing as 'standard' physiology so that 'standard values' of physiological parameters should be treated with caution and not regarded as fact. Secondly, that by studying physiology (or any science) during changing circumstances and at the extremities of normality, one can learn a lot about mechanisms which operate under more normal conditions.

May 1993   R.M.C.
Manchester   J.M.W.

CONTENTS

CONTRIBUTORS

R.M. Case, D.E. Evans, H.O. Garland, R. Green,
E.C. Griffiths, D.S. Minors, and J.M. Waterhouse, School
of Biological Sciences, University of Manchester, Oxford
Road, Manchester, M13 9PT.

R.A. Little, North Western Injury Research Centre, University
of Manchester, address as above.

C.P. Sibley, School of Biological Sciences and Department of
Child Health, University of Manchester, address as above.

1

The pregnant woman

1.1 Introduction

A woman's physiology changes during pregnancy. However, just as the physiology of the 'average 70 kg man' cannot represent all non-pregnant human beings, so there is no such thing in real life as the average pregnant woman. A large number of factors influence the degree of physiological change during pregnancy. These include the mother's age, ethnic origin and environment, the number of fetuses she is carrying, the number of previous pregnancies, and also the genetic make-up of the fetus and placenta. Nevertheless, for scientific understanding of pregnancy and for care of the pregnant woman it is necessary to know what the mean physiological changes are. It is these which are described in this chapter.

1.2 The demands of pregnancy

Pregnancy makes two major demands: first, the nutritional and metabolic demands of the weight gain required by the fetus and other products of conception, which also requires weight gain by the mother and, secondly, the demands of labour which, even in a normal pregnancy, cause physiological stress.

1.2.1 Growth and body weight changes in the fetus and mother

The fetus at term (40 weeks from the first day of the last menstrual period) weighs 3.5 kg on average (Fig. 1.1). However, there is considerable variation. Fetal weight is affected by maternal age (older women tend to have smaller babies), by maternal race and ethnicity (Asian, Oriental, and African women tend to have smaller babies than Europeans although this might be related somewhat to nutrition), by maternal weight (obese women tend to have bigger babies), by fetal sex (boys tend to be heavier than girls at birth), and the number of fetuses. Although, because of these factors, it is difficult to determine what the weight at birth of a normal baby should be, it is clear that this is a vital factor in determining lifetime health. Fetuses which show retarded growth *in utero* and which are born as 'small for gestational age' have six times the normal risk of neurodevelopmental handicap at 1 year of age. Epidemiological evidence also suggests that small size at birth predisposes to hypertension in adult life. Growth retardation may be due to a number of factors, not all related to the nutrition of the mother, but a major demand of pregnancy must be to ensure that an adequate nutrient supply is available to the developing fetus.

Placental growth shows a different pattern to fetal growth (Fig. 1.2) but, because of the direct relationship between net nutrient transfer from mother to fetus and placental surface area (see below), this must also be important in ensuring normal size at birth.

The maternal component of the total weight gain at term (Fig. 1.1) averages 7.7 kg and comprises increases in uterine and breast tissue, extra-cellular fluid, and fat. The uterus shows a dramatic increase in cavity volume, from 10 ml prior to pregnancy to 5 l at term. This increase in size is due mainly to stretching and hypertrophy of existing muscle cells. Initially hypertrophy is stimulated by oestrogen and possibly progesterone but after the third month it is due to the effect of the pressure exerted by the expand-ing fetus. Extracellular fluid volume is increased by almost 3 l at term. A 50 per cent plasma volume expansion accounts for approximately half of this increase (see below); the remainder is interstitial fluid. In women suffering pathological oedema[1] during pregnancy the increase in interstitial fluid alone may approach 5 l out of a total weight gain of 14.5 kg. Oedema is a normal finding in pregnancy. When it is not excessive and not accom-panied by hypertension and proteinuria, it is actually a good sign of adequate extracellular fluid expansion. Such women and their babies tend to be healthier than those who do not develop oedema. This is therefore distinguished from the excessive extracellular fluid expansion meant by

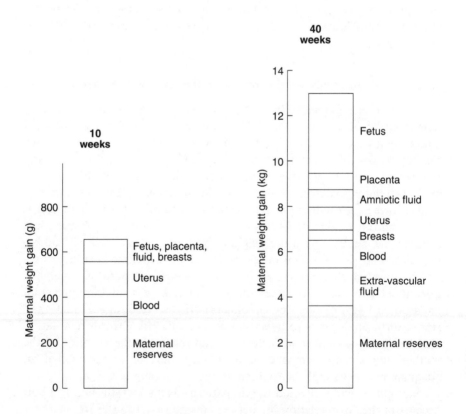

Fig. 1.1. Maternal weight gain and distribution at 10 and 40 weeks of pregnancy. Note the difference in scales.

'pathological oedema'. Including the fetus the total accumulation of water during pregnancy may be 6–8 l.

As far as the fetus is concerned, probably the most important component of the maternal weight gain is the accumulation of approximately 3 kg of fat. Maternal fat stores are laid down primarily during the first half of pregnancy and provide an energy store for the third trimester when fetal growth predominates (Figs 1.1 and 1.2).

1.2.2 Demands of labour

Labour is divided into three stages. The first stage commences when uterine contractions are of sufficient frequency, intensity, and duration to bring about dilatation of the cervix. The second stage of labour begins when dilatation of the cervix is complete and ends with delivery of the infant. The third stage of labour begins with delivery of the infant and ends with delivery of the placenta. This process requires a sustained, vigorous effort for as long as 24 h and therefore makes considerable demands of a woman's physiology. However, because of the difficulties with making measurements

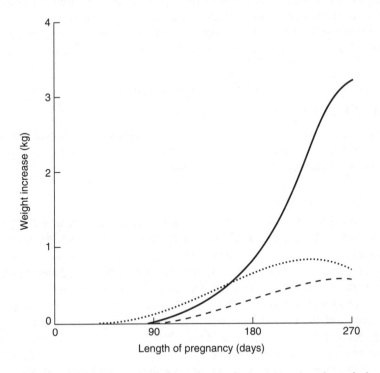

Fig. 1.2. Weight gain of the fetus (——) placenta (······) and amniotic fluid (------) throughout pregnancy. From Hytten, F. and Chamberlain, G. (1980). *Clinical physiology in obstetrics*. Blackwell, Oxford.

during this period these demands are not well documented although some generalizations may be made.

Basal cardiac output increases by 12 per cent during the first stage of labour, with each uterine contraction causing a further 35 per cent increase. Valsalvas manoeuvres and uterine contractions cause even higher and longer-lasting cardiac output increments during the second stage. Immediately after labour there is a marked rise in resting cardiac output because of increased venous return, secondary to the decreased volume of the utero-placental circulation and elimination of the uterine pressure on the inferior vena cava.

There is a considerable blood loss of approximately 600 ml on delivery of a single fetus, but which might be as much as 1 l during Caesarean section or on vaginal delivery of twins. The quantity of erythrocytes lost may equal or exceed the added volume accumulated during pregnancy (see below).

The energy demands of labour are significant and are met by the breakdown of carbohydrate. After each uterine contraction there is a significant increase in maternal lactate and metabolic acidosis is common in labour.

There is little intake of fluid during labour whilst fluid is lost through the lungs and skin and in urine. However, dehydration does not usually become too severe unless the labour lasts much longer than 24 h.

It is in the light of all these demands that the following description of the physiological changes which occur during pregnancy must be considered.

1.3 Physiological adaptations to pregnancy

1.3.1 Changes in the endocrine system

The changes in the physiology of a woman which occur during pregnancy are certainly associated with and in many systems caused by endocrine changes. A number of organs are involved.

1.3.1.1 *The placenta*

A major function of the placenta is to act as an endocrine organ. It produces both peptide and steroid hormones. The peptide hormones, human chorionic gonadotrophin (hCG) and human placental lactogen (hPL) are produced exclusively by the placenta. hCG is produced by trophoblast cells as early as the blastocyst stage and is therefore used for diagnosis of pregnancy. It is structurally similar to luteinizing hormone and functions to maintain the corpus luteum which consequently continues to produce oestrogen and progesterone during the first 3 months of pregnancy until the placenta can take over this role. These steroid hormones are essential in maintaining pregnancy. The plasma concentration of hCG peaks between 10 and 12 weeks of pregnancy and then declines to term (Fig. 1.3). The plasma concentration of hPL on the other hand continues to rise throughout pregnancy peaking near to term (Fig. 1.3). hPL is structurally similar to growth hormone and prolactin and has similar functions, namely to mobilize free fatty acids, antagonize the actions of insulin, and cause retention of potassium, nitrogen, and other minerals.

Production and secretion of progesterone and oestrogen increase throughout pregnancy (Fig. 1.3). The placenta does not have all the enzymes required to synthesize oestrogens and therefore utilizes precursors from the fetal adrenal cortex. As will be obvious from the subsequent sections these steroid hormones have a profound effect on pregnancy.

1.3.1.2 *The pituitary*

The pituitary increases in size but is not essential for pregnancy as women who have been hypophysectomized (surgical removal of the pituitary) successfully complete pregnancy. In normal women the secretion of prolactin, adrenocorticotrophic hormone (ACTH), and melanocyte-stimulating hormone is increased. Growth hormone and gonadotrophin production are reduced, the former possibly by hPL and the latter by placental steroids.

1.3.1.3 *The adrenal*

There is an increase in both total and free plasma cortisol during pregnancy. Free cortisol normally suppresses ACTH production. Therefore, the fact

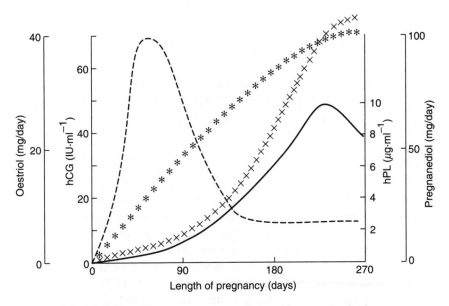

Fig. 1.3. Maternal plasma concentrations of human chorionic gonadotrophin (hCG, ------), human placental lactogen (hPL, ——), and the daily excretion rates of oestriol (xxxxx) and pregnanediol (a urinary metabolite of progesterone, *****) throughout pregnancy. From Case, R.M. (ed.) (1985). *Variations in human physiology.* Manchester University Press.

that both hormones increase suggests that the normal feedback relationship between the two is altered.

Aldosterone secretion is increased both by the natriuretic effect of progesterone and because there is also a rise in renin and angiotensin levels.

1.3.1.4 *The thyroid*

The thyroid gland enlarges during pregnancy and the production of thyroxine and tri-iodothyronine is increased. However, their free plasma concentrations are unchanged as the production of thyroid-binding proteins also increases.

1.3.1.5 *Calcium regulating hormones*

Pregnancy causes a fall in the plasma ionized calcium concentration. This results in an increase in parathyroid hormone concentrations and, in the presence of adequate vitamin D, a rise in circulating $1,25(OH)_2D_3$ concentrations. This will increase calcium absorption by the gut so as to maintain the calcium supply to the fetus (see later). Plasma calcitonin concentration rises despite the reduction in the plasma ionized calcium concentration and its cause is unknown.

1.3.2 **Changes in metabolism**

1.3.2.1 *Carbohydrates*

Carbohydrate metabolism changes characteristically during pregnancy as a result of the rise in oestrogen, progesterone, hPL, free cortisol, and prolactin concentrations. The insulin concentration also rises from the end of the first trimester through to the third trimester, although it then declines from approximately 32 weeks to term, reaching non-pregnant levels. The fasting plasma glucose concentration of a pregnant woman falls during the first trimester, it then rises between 16 and 32 weeks before falling again towards term. This latter fall is explained by the increasing use of maternal glucose for energy by both the fetus and placenta as well as the glycosuria of pregnancy. Nevertheless, in a normal human pregnancy fasting glucose concentrations are maintained in a very narrow range (4.0–4.5 mmol/l) except after meals when they rise, the more so as gestation proceeds. Furthermore, there seems to be a progressive reduction of glucose tolerance following an oral glucose load; the time taken to reach the peak plasma glucose concentration is increased and the increment in plasma glucose concentration is greater than in the non-pregnant state. This decreased glucose tolerance is due to an increase in tissue resistance to insulin possibly as a result of effects on both receptor and intracellular signalling mechanisms. Obviously the insulin-antagonizing hormones mentioned above (hPL, steroid hormones) may have a role. Diabetes mellitus may be aggravated during pregnancy. Indeed some women develop diabetes only during pregnancy (gestational diabetes) most of whom return to normal following pregnancy although in some diabetes persists. Good glycaemic control in pregnant diabetic women is very important as hyperglycaemia appears to be a major factor leading to congenital anomalies in the fetus.

1.3.2.2 *Lipids*

The plasma concentrations of free fatty acids (FFA) and glycerol fall from early to mid-pregnancy and then rise substantially towards term. This correlates with fat storage which occurs during the first half of pregnancy and fat mobilization, which occurs during the second half. Thus, the pregnant woman spares glucose for the fetus by switching over to fat as her primary energy source. Insulin normally facilitates uptake of glucose by adipose tissue and subsequent deposition of fat, but as insulin resistance increases during pregnancy the balance of fat metabolism may be switched towards fat mobilization. The rise in plasma FFA concentrations also increases fat transfer across the placenta and, thus, provides an additional substrate to the fetal liver for lipogenesis.

Plasma concentrations of cholesterol and phospholipid also increase during pregnancy. The signficance of this change is not clear but it should increase transplacental transfer of these important substrates to the fetus.

1.3.2.3 *Amino acids and proteins*

Plasma albumin concentration decreases during pregnancy as a result of the increased plasma volume. Colloid osmotic pressure is therefore lowered, contributing to the limb oedema seen in late pregnancy.

Pregnancy causes a reduction in amino acid catabolism as amino acids are used preferentially for gluconeogenesis. Plasma amino acid concentrations fall because of this increased gluconeogenesis and also because of transplacental transfer. There is also loss of amino acids in the urine (see below). The fetus uses amino acids as an energy substrate as well as for protein synthesis.

1.3.3 Changes in the gastrointestinal system

1.3.3.1 *Dietary intake*

A woman's appetite increases in pregnancy and the energy content of her diet increases by approximately 837 kJ per day. This increase is not enough to meet the specific nutritional demands of pregnancy and the difference is made up by reducing energy output, that is, the pregnant woman rests more and may be relatively listless. The stimulation of appetite may be caused by a central action of progesterone and the decrease in plasma glucose concentrations in early pregnancy.

Many pregnant women report cravings for particular foods. These foods often have strong flavours and the craving may be related to a dulling of the taste buds. Pica, an abnormal craving for unusual substances such as coal, soap, rubber bands, etc., is part of the mythology of pregnancy; its actual incidence may be very low. A distaste for particular foods may also appear in pregnancy.

Pregnant women often also have an increased thirst. This may be caused by the raised concentrations of prolactin and angiotensin, both of which are dipsogenic in animals. The enhanced fluid intake probably contributes to the water retention and increased plasma volume typical of pregnancy.

Two dietary constituents of particular importance during pregnancy are calcium and iron. Fetal calcium requirements during the third trimester reach 0.3 g/day as its skeleton becomes calcified. This amount of calcium is approximately half the recommended dietary intake of the non-pregnant woman so that pregnant women are encouraged to increase their calcium intake by approximately 70 per cent. Maternal plasma calcium concentration is lower during pregnancy and this brings the calcitropic hormones, PTH and $1,25(OH)_2D_3$, into play. Together they enhance absorption of calcium in the duodenum and reduce urinary calcium losses.

The iron content of a normal non-pregnant woman is approximately 2 g but may be as little as 0.3 g, whereas the iron requirement of normal pregnancy is approximately 1 g. The pregnant woman therefore may need supplemental iron. The sources of iron requirement and sites of loss are shown in Fig. 1.4.

1.3.3.2 *Gastrointestinal organs*

The mouth. The major change in pregnancy appears to be to the gums which often become swollen and spongy and bleed more easily. There is an increased incidence of gingivitis and of dental caries.

The oesophagus. Gastro-oesophageal acid reflux, leading to dyspepsia and heartburn, occurs in up to 70 per cent of women particularly in the third trimester. Normally gastro-oesophageal reflux due to a rise in intragastric pressure is prevented by an adaptive rise in lower oesophageal sphincter pressure. In pregnancy there is a failure of this adaptive rise, perhaps due to the influence of progesterone and oestrogen and this can lead to reflux.

The stomach. Gastric acid secretion is reduced in pregnancy and this may be part of the reason for the reduced incidence of peptic ulcers. However, this reduction in ulcers may also result from the healthier diet, increased food intake, a less stressful life in general, and regular medical supervision.

Gastric tone and motility are reduced in pregnant women. This leads to a slowing of gastric emptying and the amount of food left in the stomach at any given time increases. Nausea and vomiting occur in 50–85 per cent of pregnancies but the underlying causes are not understood.

The intestine. There is no evidence in women of the increase in intestinal size seen in small mammals during pregnancy. As noted above calcium absorption in the duodenum increases under the influence of 1,25 $(OH)_2D_3$ and there is also an increase in the percentage of iron absorbed from an oral dose. Intestinal propulsion is reduced and the consequently raised transit time for food improves the efficiency of digestion and absorption. The smooth muscle of the colon also relaxes and this can lead to constipation. This constipation in pregnancy might also be due to an increase in the absorption of water from the colon. Angiotensin and aldosterone have both been implicated by animal experiments in this increased water absorption as has prolactin.

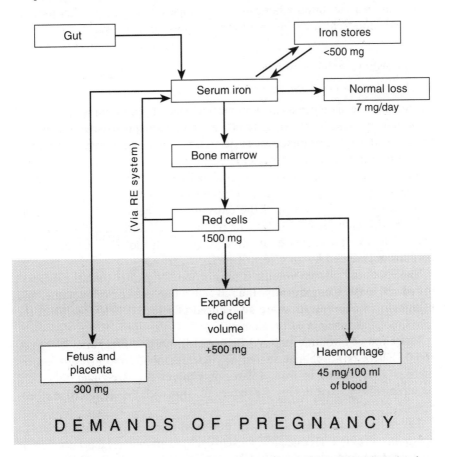

Fig. 1.4. The iron requirements of normal pregnancy. From Pritchard, J.A. *et al.* (1985). *Williams obstetrics.* Appleton-Century-Crofts, Norwalk, CT, USA.

The generalized decrease in the tone and motility of the gastrointestinal tract during pregnancy is generally ascribed to the effect of progesterone on smooth muscle. However, gut hormones also play a role as the plasma concentration of motilin, which normally stimulates gastrointestinal smooth muscle, decreases during pregnancy and that of enteroglucagon, which normally slows intestinal transit, increases.

The liver and gall bladder. Some hepatic function tests yield different results in pregnancy. Alkaline phosphatase activity in serum doubles, partially because the placenta produces a heat stable alkaline phosphatase isoform. Serum albumin and cholinesterase concentrations fall but leucine aminopeptidase activity increases due to the appearance of a pregnancy-specific enzyme. These changes are in the same direction as those observed in hepatic disease.

The gall bladder has the same muscular sluggishness seen in other parts of the gastrointestinal tract; pregnancy predisposes to gallstones.

1.3.4 Cardiovascular changes

1.3.4.1 *Blood volume and its components*

In normal pregnancy plasma volume increases by approximately 43 per cent. This increase is related to fetal mass and may approach 90 per cent in women with triplets or quadruplets. It results from an enhanced fluid intake, reduced output, and possibly a shift between body fluid compartments.

Red cell mass (total volume of red cells in the circulation) normally increases by 17–25 per cent during pregnancy. Like plasma volume, this increase varies with the size of the fetus and may be three times greater in women with multiple births. It is the result of enhanced red cell production which follows an increase in circulating erythropoietin concentration, perhaps augmented by an effect of hPL.

The enhanced plasma volume is proportionally greater than the increase in red cell mass. Consequently, the red cell count, packed cell volume, and haemoglobin concentration are all reduced (Table 1.1). This results in the 'physiological anaemia of pregnancy'.

Mean red cell volume (m.c.v.) increases in normal pregnancy by up to 100 fl. There is no change in red cell haemoglobin concentration unless there is a deficiency in iron, folate, or vitamin B_{12}. Iron and folic acid requirements increase during pregnancy to cope with the enhanced erythropoiesis.

The total white cell count rises during the third trimester of human pregnancy (Table 1.1), due almost exclusively to an increased production of neutrophils which comprise the largest fraction of the total leukocyte population. This increased production of neutrophils may be stimulated by the rising oestrogen concentration. Other white cell counts remain steady or

Table 1.1. Some haematological indices in non-pregnant and pregnant women in the third trimester

Index	Non-pregnant	Pregnant
Red cell count (cells/litre)	4.7×10^{12}	3.8×10^{12}
Packed cell volume (%)	42	33
Haemoglobin concentration (g/100 ml)	14	11.5
White cell count (cells/litre)	9×10^9	11×10^9

fall as gestation proceeds. Lymphocyte function and cellular immunity are suppressed, possibly by oestrogen, hCG, and prolactin. This helps combat fetal rejection but will, at the same time, render the mother more susceptible to infection. Indeed, there is an increased incidence of influenza, rubella, and hepatitis in pregnancy.

1.3.4.2 *Haemostasis*

There are changes in the components of the normal haemostatic mechanism during pregnancy. There is a decrease in platelet count during the third trimester, although there appears to be no change in their lifespan. There are marked changes, both increases and decreases, in the concentrations of the components of the coagulation and fibrinolytic systems, occurring as early as the second month of pregnancy.

Some of these alterations can be mimicked by the administration of contraceptives containing oestrogen and progesterone to non-pregnant women. These hormones may therefore be of importance in bringing about the normal pregnancy-induced changes.

At the time of placental separation from the uterus the normal placental blood flow of approximately 500 ml/min must be stopped within seconds if a major haemorrhage is to be avoided. Part of the haemostasis is brought about by myometrial contraction substantially reducing this blood flow. Coagulation times are not different between pregnant and non-pregnant women but the general increase in coagulation factors provides an important reserve for the haemostasis which occurs both during and after placental separation.

1.3.4.3 *Arterial blood pressure and its determinants*

Both systolic and diastolic blood pressures fall during the first trimester (Fig. 1.5). Both then rise again towards term. The effect of posture on blood pressure is even more marked in pregnant women than it is normally. In the supine position in late pregnancy, the uterus and its contents compress the vena cava which reduces venous return. Reflex vasoconstriction may maintain arterial blood pressure in this situation but, in one study of a 100 women 47 per cent had a fall in systolic pressure of 10 per cent and 10 of them experienced a 30 per cent or greater fall. This 'supine hypotension' may cause restlessness, faintness, hyperpnoea, and pallor. Poor venous return in late pregnancy can also lead to oedema in the lower leg, varicose veins, and haemorrhoids.

Cardiac output increases by approximately 40 per cent during the first trimester, because of an increase in both heart rate (from 70 to 85 beats/min) and stroke volume (from 60 to 70 ml). As arterial pressure falls despite the rise in cardiac output it follows that there must be a marked fall in peripheral resistance. In the first trimester this probably results from a decreased

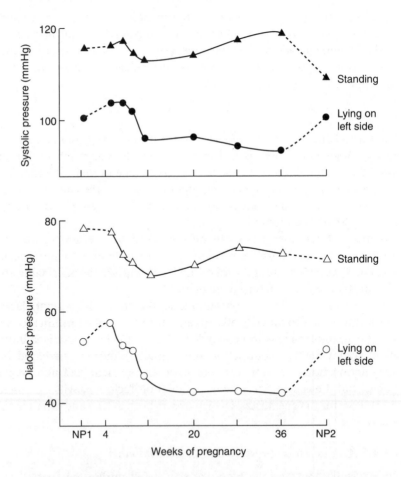

Fig. 1.5. Mean systolic and diastolic pressures of 10 women measured standing or lying before conception (NP1), during pregnancy and 6 weeks after delivery (NP2). From Redman, C. and De Swiet, M. (ed.) (1989). *Medical disorders in obstetric practice*. Blackwell, Oxford.

responsiveness of arteriolar smooth muscle to the vasoconstrictor actions of angiotensin II. Later on in pregnancy other factors might also reduce peripheral resistance including the opening of the uteroplacental circulation and the inhibitory effects of oestrogen and progesterone on arteriolar smooth muscle tone.

1.3.4.4 *Regional blood flow*

Much of the increased cardiac output is directed to the uteroplacental circulation whose blood flow increases 10-fold to approximately 750 ml/min at term. There is also an increased blood flow to the skin (which helps heat dissipation), to the breasts, and to the gastrointestinal tract. Renal blood flow increases by up to 80 per cent in the first trimester but may then fall towards term.

1.3.5 Changes in the respiratory system

Resting oxygen consumption by the end of pregnancy is 30–40 ml/min above the non-pregnant value of 220 ml/min, an increase of approximately 15 per cent. Most of this is due to fetal oxygen consumption (Fig. 1.6). The increased oxygen demand is more than met by the increased red cell mass

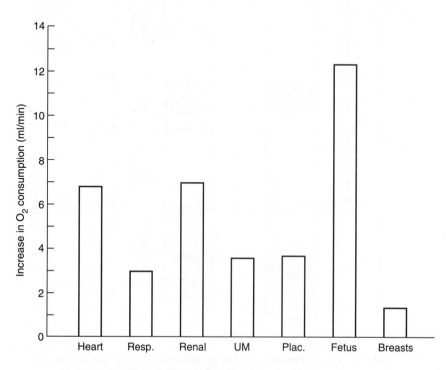

Fig. 1.6. Distribution of the increased oxygen consumption by term to various tissues. Resp. = respiration; UM = uterine muscle; Plac. = placenta.

described above (which results in an increase in the total oxygen carrying capacity of the blood) and by a 40 per cent increase in minute ventilation from 7.5 to 10.5 l/min. This change in ventilation is due solely to an increase in tidal volume (Fig. 1.7)—respiratory rate is unaltered—and probably results from a direct effect of progesterone on the respiratory centre. This causes a raised sensitivity to CO_2 so that whereas in the non-pregnant state ventilation increases by 1.5 l/min per kPa rise in PCO_2, in pregnancy it increases by 6 l/min for the same PCO_2 change.

There are marked changes in the configuration of the chest which alter lung volumes (Fig. 1.7). The lower ribs of pregnant women flare, a change which does not always recover after pregnancy, the subcostal angle increases and the transverse diameter of the chest increases by approximately 2 cm. The height of the diaphragm rises by a maximum of 4 cm but, contrary to expectation, diaphragmatic excursion is not restricted by pregnancy and is

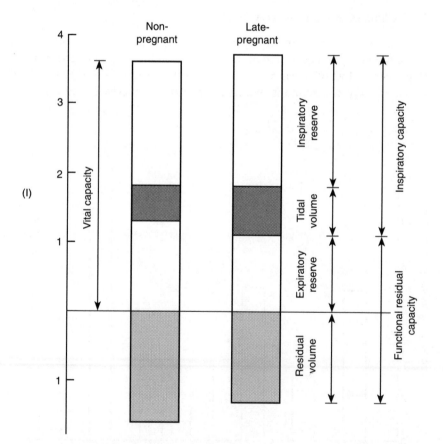

Fig. 1.7. Lung volumes in non-pregnant and late pregnant women. From Hytten, F. and Chamberlain, G. (1980). *Clinical physiology in obstetrics.* Blackwell, Oxford.

in fact increased by 1–2 cm as follows from the hyperventilation described above.

As determined by measurement of forced expiratory volume in one second (FEV_1) and peak expiratory flow rate, airway resistance is not altered by pregnancy. Pulmonary diffusing capacity, as measured using carbon monoxide, is decreased, possibly because of the decreased haemoglobin concentration (physiological anaemia) or an effect of oestrogen on the alveolar capillary wall. However, this reduced diffusing capacity is offset by a more efficient distribution of gas in the lungs and a higher alveolar PO_2 resulting from the increase in ventilation.

Becuase of the shape of the haemoglobin dissociation curve, the increase in alveolar PO_2 has little effect on haemoglobin saturation although there may be an increase in arterial PO_2. The increased ventilation decreases both alveolar and arterial PCO_2 from 5.3 to 4.0 kPa. Plasma bicarbonate decreases by an equivalent amount in order to keep the pH constant at the non-pregnant value. This results in a decrease in maternal plasma osmolarity and a resetting of the osmoreceptors in order to avoid a diuresis.

As the net rate of fetomaternal CO_2 diffusion across the placenta is determined by its concentration gradient (see below), the decreased PCO_2 of maternal blood will assist CO_2 excretion from the fetus.

Labour and parturition clearly alter normal respiratory function but the difficulties with making measurements during this period mean that these have not been quantified.

1.3.6 Changes in renal function

1.3.6.1 *Anatomy*

The kidneys generally enlarge during pregnancy; renal length may increase by approximately 1 cm. Ultrasound studies suggest that renal parenchymal volumes increase as a result of increased intrarenal fluid. The calyces, renal pelvis, and ureters all markedly dilate.

1.3.6.2 *Glomerular filtration rate (GFR) and effective renal plasma flow (ERPF)*

Both GFR and ERPF, measured by inulin and PAH (para-amino hippuric acid) clearances respectively, increase by up to 50 per cent, the initial rises occurring early in the first trimester (Fig. 1.8). The rise in GFR means that the plasma concentrations of creatinine and urea, whose production does not change during pregnancy, tend to fall.

The reason for the rise in GFR is not completely clear but probably reflects the increased renal plasma flow. However, the cause of the rise in ERPF is not understood. It may be related to the increased plasma volume. However, increases in the circulating concentrations of steroid hormones such as aldosterone, desoxycorticosterone, progesterone, and cortisol and of parathyroid hormone, hPL, and hCG may also have an effect.

1.3.6.3 *The kidney and fluid volume regulation*

As noted earlier, of the mean 12.5 kg body weight increase of a pregnant woman, approximately 6–8 l is water. Although there is increased fluid intake, renal control of salt and water output is also clearly an important factor in this fluid retention. The increase in GFR noted above will result in something like an extra 12 mol of sodium being filtered. In order to prevent this potentially catastrophic loss tubular sodium and water reabsorption is increased. This is achieved so efficiently that, coupled with the increased intake of food, it leads to a retention of approximately 950 mmol of sodium during pregnancy. The energy required for this increased renal reabsorption of sodium contributes significantly to the metabolic cost of pregnancy.

The mechanisms responsible for the increased reabsorption of sodium are not certain although stimulation of the renin–angiotensin–aldosterone system must contribute. These mechanisms must offset the natriuretic

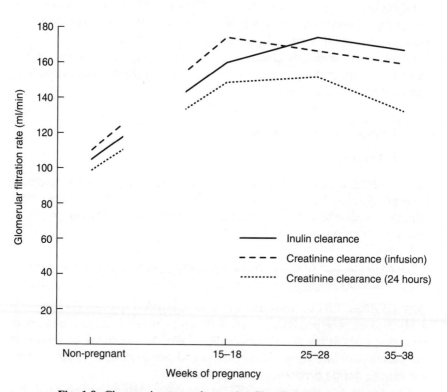

Fig. 1.8. Changes in mean glomerular filtration rate during pregnancy as measured by three different methods. From Davison, J. and De Swiet, M. (ed.) (1989). *Medical disorders in obstetric practice.* Blackwell, Oxford.

effects of progesterone and some other hormones whose secretion is increased, as well as the effects of a raised GFR.

Soon after conception a woman's plasma osmolality falls by approximately 10 mosmol/kg H_2O. Normally this would lead to a fall in antidiuretic hormone (ADH) secretion and a diuresis. This does not happen in the pregnant woman which suggests that her osmoreceptors are somehow 'reset' to a lower value. In fact the ability to excrete a water load does decline during the third trimester. Clearly this also contributes to the water gains of pregnancy.

1.3.6.4 *Renal handling of other solutes*

Glycosuria is a common feature of normal human pregnancy, starting within 6 weeks of the last menstrual period. The excretion of fructose, lactose, ribose, and xylose also increase. The most likely cause of the glycosuria is the increase in GFR but a diminished ability of the proximal and possibly distal tubule to reabsorb glucose might also contribute.

Excretion of most amino acids also increases and may reach up to 2 g/day. The cause is unknown but may reflect decreased tubular reabsorption rather than increased GFR as plasma amino acid concentrations generally fall. This loss of amino acids may be nutritionally significant when protein intake is suboptimal.

The excretion of water-soluble vitamins (nicotinic acid, ascorbic acid, and folate) increases during pregnancy and, as for amino acids, may reflect decreased tubular reabsorption.

Although a raised aldosterone concentration, amongst other factors, might be expected to increase potassium excretion during pregnancy, there is in fact a retention of approximately 350 mmol. As in men kaliuresis can be abolished by intramuscular administration of progesterone, it is thought that this hormone might be responsible for the pregnancy-induced conservation of potassium in women.

1.3.7 **The placenta in maternofetal exchange**

The placenta, vital for normal fetal growth and development, of necessity affects the physiology of the pregnant woman. It has three main functions: it is an important endocrine organ of pregnancy (see above), it protects the fetal allograft from attack by the maternal immune system, and it is the interface between maternal and fetal plasma across which maternofetal transfer of nutrients and waste products occurs. This latter function is considered in this section.

1.3.7.1 *General considerations*

The placenta shows the greatest morphological diversity across species of any mammalian organ and its physiological characteristics undoubtedly show similar diversity. An example of this diversity is shown in Fig. 1.9. The pig and sheep placentas have four continuous cell layers separating maternal and fetal plasma whereas the human placenta only has two. Not surprisingly, therefore, the permeability of the sheep placenta to extra-cellular space markers, such as mannitol, is at least 20 times lower than that for the human. These differences make it even more difficult than normal to extrapolate from one species to another and the following is therefore concerned only with the human placenta.

The two cell layers separating maternal and fetal blood in the human placenta are the syncytiotrophoblast (probably the main barrier to materno-fetal exchange) and the fetal capillary endothelium (Fig. 1.9). Solutes may cross these cell layers by passive diffusion, carrier mediated transport, and endocytosis/exocytosis.

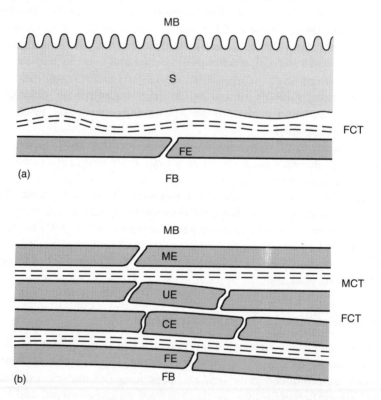

Fig. 1.9. Diagrammatic representation of two histologically defined types of placenta. (a) Haemochorial placenta as in the human. (b) Epithelio-chorial placenta as in the pig. MB, maternal blood; FB, fetal blood; S, syncytiotrophoblast cell layer; FCT, fetal connective tissue; FE, fetal capillary endothelium; ME, maternal capillary endothelium; MCT, maternal connective tissue; UE, uterine epithelium; CE, chorionic epithelium. From Sibley, C.P. and Boyd, R.D.H. (1992) (see Further reading list).

Passive diffusion. Ficks Law of Diffusion related to placental exchange may be stated as

$$J = \frac{AD}{l} (C_m - C_f)$$

where J is the rate of transfer (mol/s), A is the surface area available for exchange (m²), D is the diffusion coefficient of the solute in question (m²/s), l is the path length or thickness of the barrier (m) and $(C_m - C_f)$ is the concentration gradient between maternal and fetal plasma (mol/l).

The term AD/l represents placental 'permeability' for the solute in question and in general is high for hydrophobic solutes and low for hydrophilic solutes. The high permeability of hydrophobic solutes means that their rate of transfer depends more on their delivery to the site of exchange (effectively maternal and fetal blood flow) than on their rate of diffusion across the placenta. Their transfer is therefore said to be flow-limited. The reverse is true for hydrophilic solutes, whose rate of diffusion is more limiting for transfer than is the rate of delivery and are therefore said to be diffusion- or membrane-limited. This is shown diagrammatically in Fig. 1.10. The flow limitation of hydrophobic solutes means that their rate of transfer will also be dependent on the geometric arrangement of maternal and fetal circulations. Maternal blood spurts in a fountain-like manner into the intervillous space of the human placenta and therefore the arrangement of the maternal and fetal circulations is not as efficient for exchange as a countercurrent system (where blood flows in the opposite direction in the two circulations) would be but is more efficient than a concurrent system (where blood flows in the same direction in the two circulations) would be.

For charged species the electrical gradient or potential difference (p.d.) across the syncytiotrophoblast will also have an important effect on diffusion. The existence or otherwise of such a p.d. has been controversial but the latest estimates using microelectrode impalements of term placenta suggest it is approximately 4 mV, fetal side negative. This would thus increase the rate of transfer of positively charged species towards the fetus but retard negatively charged ones.

Carrier-mediated transport. Transcellular transport across the syncytiotrophoblast requires two transport proteins, one in the maternal-facing plasma membrane and one in the fetal-facing plasma membrane. One of these may be a channel rather than a carrier. This is described more fully in considering calcium and amino acid transport below.

Endocytosis/exocytosis. Large, usually protein, molecules may gain access into the cell by fluid phase endocytosis in which the plasma membrane invaginates to engulf solute and water in the extracellular space. In receptor-mediated endocytosis the solute binds to specific receptors on the plasma membrane in the area which eventually invaginates. These are usually in regions called coated pits and the vesicle of the plasma membrane which becomes internalized is called a coated vesicle. Vesicles may eventually fuse with the opposite pole of the cell and expel their contents by exocytosis thus bringing about transfer. The syncytiotrophoblast of the human placenta is well endowed with coated pits and vesicles and so this may well be a mechanism of maternofetal transfer used for large molecules such as immunoglobulin G.

1.3.7.2 *Some specific examples of transported molecules*

Oxygen and carbon dioxide. These gases are small hydrophobic molecules which therefore have a high permeability and are transferred by flow-limited passive diffusion. The concentration gradients between maternal

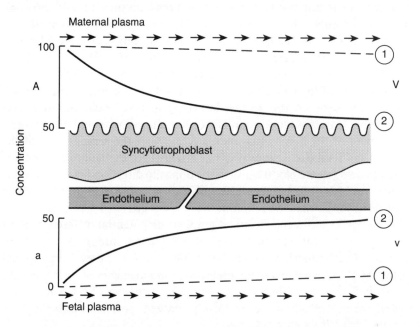

Fig. 1.10. Diagrammatic representation of flow limitation and membrane limitation. The expected plasma concentration profiles of two substances (1 and 2) in the maternal and fetal circulations of a haemochorial placenta. Plasma flows from the arterial end (A and a) to the venous end (V and v) of the exchange area. For simplicity the flows in the two compartments are shown as concurrent and are of equal magnitude. Substance 1 is hydrophilic and is membrane-limited; maternal and fetal concentrations never approach each other and the rate of delivery is not limiting. Substance 2 is small and hydrophobic and is flow-limited; the maternal and fetal concentrations approach each other before the end of the exchange area and the amount transferred depends on the rate of delivery. From Sibley, C.P. and Boyd, R.D.H. *In* Clarke, J.R. (1988). *Oxford reviews of reproductive biology,* vol. 10. Oxford University Press.

and fetal plasma allow this; maternal plasma PO_2 is 12.0 kPa while that in fetal plasma is 3.0–5.0 kPa. The equivalent values for carbon dioxide are 3.5–4.0 and 5.0–5.5 kPa respectively. Oxygen transfer is aided by the higher affinity of fetal haemoglobin for oxygen as compared with adult haemoglobin and by the Bohr effect, resulting from the diffusion of carbon dioxide out of the fetal plasma. The flow limitation to oxygen diffusion may be clinically important as any condition which leads to reduced placental blood flow, such as maternal hypertension or umbilical cord compression during delivery, will reduce oxygen transfer and may result in fetal asphyxia.

Sodium and chloride. The transfer of these two ions across the human placenta is probably mainly by membrane-limited passive diffusion. However, transport proteins for both ions have been found in maternal-facing and fetal-facing plasma membranes of the syncytiotrophoblast. As regards sodium, an Na^+/H^+ exchanger, an Na^+ and phosphate co-transporter, and at least three Na^+ and amino acid co-transporters are present in the maternal-facing plasma membrane and Na^+, K^+ ATPase is found in the fetal-facing membrane. As regards chloride, a chloride channel is found in the maternal-facing plasma membrane and an anion exchanger is found in both maternal-facing and fetal-facing plasma membranes. Therefore, carrier-mediated transport may have a role in the transfer of both ions, particularly for chloride for which there is an adverse electrical gradient.

Calcium. The ionized calcium concentrations in maternal and fetal plasma are approximately 1.12 and 1.41 mM respectively. Net transfer to the fetus is therefore by active carrier-mediated transport. The ionized calcium concentration in syncytiotrophoblast cytosol is approximately 10^{-7} M. By analogy with the calcium transport mechanism across the duodenum, the ion may leak into the syncytiotrophoblast from the maternal plasma down its electrochemical gradient possibly utilizing a channel. In order to maintain a low cytosolic calcium concentration, the ion is probably bound to a calcium-binding protein in the cell before being pumped out into the fetal plasma against the concentration gradient by a high affinity Ca-ATPase. Such a leak/pump system would seem an elegant mechanism for materno-fetal transfer but as yet there is only firm evidence in the human placenta for the high affinity Ca-ATPase.

Iron. Transferrin binds iron in plasma. This high molecular weight complex is taken up by the maternal facing plasma membrane of the syncytiotrophoblast via receptor-mediated endocytosis. Within the cell, the iron is dissociated from transferrin and may then be stored attached to another protein, ferritin, or transferred to the fetal plasma by a mechanism which is as yet uncertain.

Glucose. The transfer of glucose across the human placenta is by facilitated diffusion using two carriers, one in the maternal-facing membrane and one in the fetal-facing membrane. Both have quite low affinities so that the rate of net transfer to the fetus is essentially dependent on the maternofetal concentration gradient (hence, the importance of maintaining maternal plasma glucose concentrations—see above). However, the placenta also requires glucose and this complicates the seemingly simple picture of maternofetal exchange.

Amino acids. In general terms amino acids are actively transported between mother and fetus. Like most other organs the placenta has a range of transporter proteins specific to different classes of amino acid viz. anionic, cationic, and neutral amino acids. Within the latter class there are further divisions of transporter specificity. In general, cytosolic concentrations of amino acids in the syncytiotrophoblast are higher than in either maternal or fetal plasma and they are said to be transported by a pump/leak system (cf. Ca^{2+}, leak/pump). For small neutral amino acids such as alanine the pump is an Na^+-dependent carrier in the maternal-facing plasma membrane which utilizes the Na^+ gradient set up by Na^+,K^+ ATPase. However, other amino acids such as leucine utilize an Na^+-independent carrier in this plasma membrane; it is not yet certain how their transport into the cell against a concentration gradient is energized. At the basal membrane there are transport proteins which can act as 'leak' carriers for amino acid transport into fetal plasma. Na^+-dependent carriers are also found in the basal membrane; whilst the role of these is not well understood, they may be involved in transporting amino acids from fetal plasma into the syncytiotrophoblast under certain conditions. The latter serves to emphasize that, as with glucose, amino acid metabolic interactions between mother, placenta, and fetus during pregnancy are complex.

Immunoglobulin. The fetus attains a certain degree of passive immunity whilst *in utero* by transfer of immunoglobulins of the gamma class (IgG) across the placenta. IgGs are high molecular weight proteins whose uptake at the maternal-facing plasma membrane of the syncytiotrophoblast is by receptor-mediated endocytosis. It is generally presumed that IgG is released from the syncytiotrophoblast following exocytosis of the vesicle. However, the actual evidence for this is currently not strong.

Drugs. Small hydrophobic compounds are rapidly transferred by flow-limited passive diffusion. Thus, if alcohol intake during pregnancy is excessive a large amount will be transferred to the fetus and may result in growth retardation. The diffusion of hydrophilic drugs on the other hand is membrane-limited and slower but, nevertheless, may still be sufficient to be potentially dangerous to the fetus.

Water. It follows from the high proportion of water in the fetus that its transfer rate across the placenta must be extremely high. However, its mechanism of transfer is poorly, if at all, understood other than the general observation that it is driven by osmotic and hydrostatic pressure gradients between maternal and fetal plasma.

1.3.7.3 *Placental insufficiency*

In some pregnancies the placenta may fail to function normally thus causing fetal growth retardation and even intrauterine death. The cause(s) of 'placental insufficiency' are largely unknown but may be due to fetal or maternal factors. A failure of the placenta to implant adequately may lead to uteroplacental blood flow becoming restricted. This may also result from maternal hypertension (pre-eclampsia or essential hypertension) due to blockage and constriction of the spiral arteries. Such conditions will obviously reduce the transfer of flow-limited solutes such as oxygen. Recent information suggests that some cases of poor growth *in utero* are associated with reduced amino acid transport by the placenta. Placental transfer may also be inadequate in multiple pregnancies. If growth retardation is severe the baby may have to be delivered prematurely otherwise death *in utero* may occur.

1.4 Parturition

The primary events causing delivery of the baby are the development of rhythmic and co-ordinated contractions of the uterine muscle (myometrium) and dilatation of the cervix. Parturition has to occur at a time when the fetus has reached a stage of development when it is capable of independent life, approximately 40 weeks in women and, thus, has to be carefully regulated physiologically. However, up to 9 per cent of all deliveries in the UK and North America occur preterm (before 37 completed weeks of gestation). In premature births, the risk of problems is directly related to the degree of prematurity.

The activity of the myometrium at term is quite different from that earlier in pregnancy. In women the frequency of contractions increases from approximately 0.3/h at 25 weeks to 2.3/h at 40 weeks. The key question is: what causes this increased activity and signals the start of parturition at the correct time? This question has been most completely answered in the sheep, where increased activity of the fetal hypothalamus–pituitary–adrenal cortex–placenta axis is pivotal. The main feature is a rise in cortisol production by the fetal adrenal which stimulates an increased production of oestrogen and a reduced production of progesterone by the placenta. This increase in the ratio of oestrogen to progesterone may then result in increased production of prostaglandins from the placenta, which in turn stimulates uterine activity and parturition. This elegant scheme is not directly applicable to women, as evidenced by the fact that anencephalic babies deliver at the same time as normal babies. In humans the key signals are therefore still obscure. However, some of the features of the sheep model may still be of importance particularly with reference to the prostaglandins. The precise role of oxytocin in parturition in women is unclear. Although it certainly stimulates uterine contractility (and is used to induce labour), it seems unlikely that it initiates parturition.

The cervix is important as a seal to maintain human pregnancy. It undergoes major changes during pregnancy such that its vascularization, mass, and water content increase whilst the mass and organization of its collagen and dermatan sulphate decrease. The changes in the cervix which allow delivery are profound, involving a remodelling of the cervical matrix with new collagen and proteoglycan synthesis. They probably began before the onset of labour and are not the direct result of myometrial contractions.

1.5 The puerperium

This is literally defined as the period of confinement during and just after birth but it has come to include the subsequent weeks during which the reproductive tract returns to the non-pregnant state. The changes in a woman's physiology which occurred during pregnancy reverse quite rapidly during this period. By approximately 6 weeks after delivery the non-nursing mother's pituitary–ovarian synchrony will have returned such that ovulation is possible and the reproductive tract will have returned anatomically to the non-pregnant state. Most women lose approximately 2 kg in weight during the first 10 days after delivery, so beginning to reverse the fluid gain of pregnancy. Cardiac output also returns to the non-pregnant level very soon after delivery.

Further reading

Brudenell, M. and Doddridge, M. (1989). *Diabetic pregnancy*. Churchill Livingstone, London.

Challis, J.R.G. and Olson, D.M. (1988). Parturition. In *The physiology of reproduction*, Vol. 2, (ed. E. Knobil, J.D. Neil), pp. 2177–216. Raven Press, New York.

De Swiet, M. (ed.) (1989). *Medical disorders in obstetric practice*. Blackwell, Oxford.

Hytten, F. and Chamberlain, G. (ed.) (1980). *Clinical physiology in obstetrics*. Blackwell, Oxford.

Pritchard, J.A., MacDonald, P.C., and Gant, N.F. (1985). *Williams obstetrics*. Appleton-Century-Crofts, Norwalk, CT.

Sibley, C.P. and Boyd, R.D.H. (1992). Mechanisms of transfer across the human placenta. In *Fetal and neonatal physiology*, (ed. R.A. Polin, W.W. Fox), pp. 62–74. W.B. Saunders, Philadelphia.

Acknowledgements

I am very grateful to Drs A. Kuruvilla, D. Mahendran, and M. Hollingsworth for helpful discussion and comments on this chapter.

2

The fetus and the neonate

2.1 Introduction

Prior to conception the fetus relies on its mother for oxygen supply, nutrition, excretion, homeostasis, and temperature regulation. Many of these functions are performed by the placenta, a specialized organ not found in the newborn (see Chapter 1). This chapter discusses the differences between the fetus, the neonate, and the adult and aims to show how final adult function is achieved. Although many parents feel that offspring are still dependent at 20 or 25 years of age, we shall assume that independent life begins at birth. Some problems of the neonate are also considered but these should be regarded as illustrative, not all embracing.

2.2 The cardiovascular system

2.2.1 Circulation in the fetus

Circulation in the fetus is shown in Fig. 2.1. The lungs are non-functional until birth and blood flow is diverted away from them. In addition, there is a large blood flow to the placenta which has to supply oxygen, nutrients, and acts as the excretory organ.

Because of the embryological development of the heart there is a potential communication between the right and left atria—the foramen ovale. A flap valve, the septum secundum, closes this on the left atrial side, so when pressure in the left atrium is higher than the right, there is effective closure. When pressure is higher in the right atrium than in the left, there is a communication channel between the two. In the fetus, blood flow to the right atrium is high because it receives the returning blood from the body plus that from the placenta and this results in a high right atrial pressure. Since blood is shunted from the lungs the flow to the left atrium is low resulting in low pressure and a patent foramen ovale. The strict anatomical relationships (see Fig. 2.2) result in the stream of blood from the inferior vena cava being directed against the interatrial septum and so most of the shunted blood comes from this stream, while the blood from the superior vena cava passes mainly to the right ventricle. Because the lungs are collapsed with constriction of the pulmonary vasculature, the pressure in the pulmonary circulation is high. This has two consequences: the right ventricular wall when compared with the left ventricular wall is proportionately much thicker than in the adult (in fact it is about the same thickness as the left) and there is a greater tendency for blood to flow from the pulmonary circulation to the systemic circulation if any connections exist.

Developmentally there is a major connection between the pulmonary artery and the aorta via the ductus arteriosus, a wide muscular walled channel. Because of the high pressure in the pulmonary circulation and the relatively low pressure in the systemic circulation (due to the low resistance circulation of the placenta) most of the blood ejected by the right ventricle

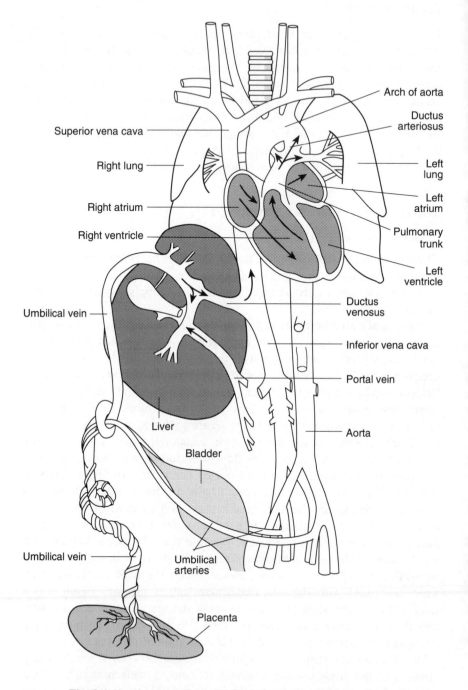

Fig. 2.1. A scheme to show the fetal circulation. Redrawn from *Grays Anatomy* (ed. Johnston, T.B., Davies, D.V., and Davies, F.), 32nd edn. p. 724. Churchill Livingstone, Edinburgh.

finds its way into the systemic circulation and only approximately 15 per cent goes to the lungs. The small fraction of blood from the right ventricle which passes to the lungs is returned via the pulmonary veins to the left atrium where it meets the large amount delivered through the foramen ovale and passes via the mitral valve into the left ventricle for distribution to the systemic circulation.

The output from the left ventricle is distributed to the head and upper limbs and it is then joined by the blood from the ductus arteriosus. This is then distributed via the descending aorta to all the abdominal organs, the body wall, and the lower limbs. Special mention must be made of the blood supply to the gastrointestinal tract which is small, as a result of the non-functional nature of the tract. All the venous drainage enters the liver at the porta hepatis, perfuses the liver with the blood derived from the hepatic artery (a branch of the coeliac axis) and passes via the hepatic veins to the inferior vena cava.

A large proportion of the blood from the descending aorta (approximately equivalent to the output from each ventricle), passes via the umbilical arteries to the placenta where oxygenation occurs. Blood passes back via the umbilical vein into the left branch of the hepatic portal vein. Here there is a shunt between the portal vein and the inferior vena cava. Approximately

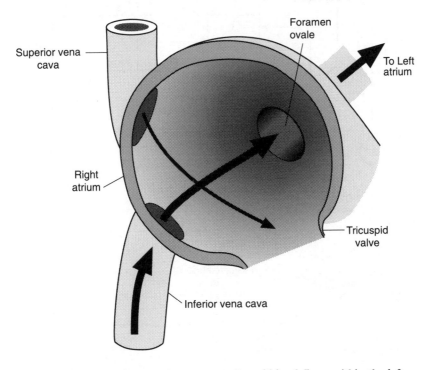

Fig. 2.2. Diagrammatic representation of blood flows within the left atrium.

40 per cent of the blood from the umbilical vein joins that from the gastro-intestinal tract and passes via the liver while the remaining 60 per cent bypasses the liver and enters the inferior vena cava directly through the ductus venosus. Blood flowing into the inferior vena cava enters the right atrium when much of it is diverted to the left atrium (see above).

Thus, there are four shunts in the fetal circulation not present in the adult, the foramen ovale, the ductus arteriosus, the placenta, and the ductus venosus. Effectively these convert the heart from two series pumps, as in the adult, to two parallel pumps.

Because of these anatomical shunts PO_2 is not the same in all parts of the arterial system. Oxygenation occurs in the placenta, and blood in the umbilical vein has the highest PO_2 in the body (see Fig. 2.3). Since only umbilical vein blood passes into the ductus venosus this also has a high concentration but further up the inferior vena cava, where it is joined by

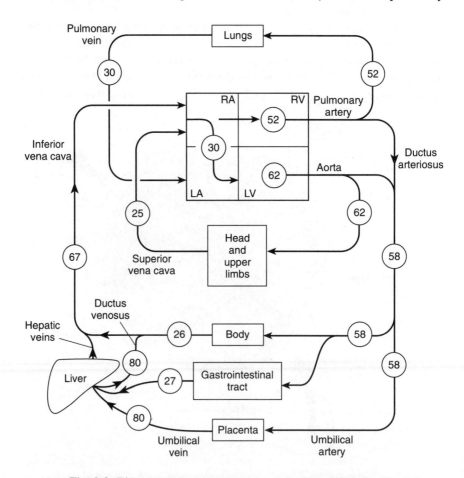

Fig. 2.3. Diagrammatic representation of the fetal circulation to show percentage haemoglobin saturation in various vessels.

deoxygenated blood from most abdominal organs and the lower limbs, the oxygen content has declined. Because some umbilical vein blood passes into the liver via the portal vein, the liver is relatively well oxygenated. Blood in the superior vena cava is deoxygenated but because there is incomplete mixing of the streams of blood from the inferior and superior vena cava, the blood which flows through the foramen ovale has a much higher oxygen content than that going into the right ventricle. Right ventricular blood going to the lungs is therefore relatively poorly oxgenated; note that the lungs and other pulmonary structures extract oxygen so the blood entering the left atrium from the pulmonary veins has a low concentration of oxygen. Since the volume of pulmonary blood is small compared to that entering via the foramen ovale, the overall drop in oxygen concentration between the inferior vena cava and left atrium is small. The anatomical arrangements ensure that the head, arms, and in particular, the coronary arteries receive this blood with a relatively high oxygenation (probably reflected in the greater relative growth of these organs when compared to the rest of the body in the fetus). The concentration of oxygen falls when aortic blood is diluted with less well oxygenated blood from the ductus arteriosus.

2.2.2 Changes in the circulation at birth

When the baby takes its first breath two major changes cause a reduction in the pulmonary vascular resistance. Firstly, the lungs are stretched mechanically and stretching of the alveoli results in stretching of the capillaries and arterioles. Secondly, when air enters the lungs PO_2 in the alveoli rises dramatically and the direct effect of this increased PO_2 on pulmonary arterioles causes vasodilation (see p. 43). Both these events result in increased blood flow and a reduction in pressure in the pulmonary artery. The pressure gradient in the fetus is now reversed and blood flows from the high pressure aorta into the lower pressure pulmonary artery, a dramatic reversal of flow.

A few minutes after this, circulation to the placenta ceases. In nature the umbilical cord is torn or bitten across and separated from the placenta. The tissue damage results in spasm of the smooth muscle of the umbilical vessels which may be intensified by the effects of circulating catecholamines or stimulation of the sympathetic nerves supplying the abdominal parts of the vessels. Together these mechanisms result in an effective clamping of the umbilical arteries and vein and blood flow ceases. In humans this mechanism is usually circumvented by the midwife or obstetrician tying off the cord. The optimum time for tying off the umbilical cord is still a matter for some debate (see p. 45). However it is caused, when placental flow ceases the general systemic resistance is raised increasing the systemic blood pressure. Because of this reduced flow there is a fall in inferior vena cava flow and the pressure in the right atrium falls. As explained above the flow in the pulmonary circulation increases and so the pressure in the left atrium rises and becomes higher than that in the right atrium. Because of this reversal of the pressure gradient the septum secundum, the flap valve over the foramen ovale is forced closed. At this stage the closure is not permanent and, indeed, in 10–15 per cent of individuals there still remains some communication even in adult life. In the majority, however, permanent closure occurs by fusion of the septum secundum with the edges of the foramen ovale. This may take 4–6 weeks.

Closure of the ductus arteriosus is also not complete at birth but functional closure occurs 10–15 h after birth. Contraction of the smooth muscle of the ductus arteriosus depends on the local increase in PO_2 that occurs. It is exquisitely sensitive to PO_2 when investigated *in vitro* and the sensitivity is increased towards the end of gestation. Prostaglandins also seem to play some role. Locally produced prostaglandins and thromboxanes as well as circulating prostaglandin E_1 and E_2 are important in maintaining patency of the ductus during fetal life, though whether this is via endothelial-derived relaxing factor or nitric oxide is not yet known. Prostaglandin inhibitors can be used to enhance closure in difficult cases and surgery for patent ductus is beginning to be a thing of the past. The increased concentration of circulating catecholamines present at birth may help in the immediate closure. Final closure of the ductus arteriosus by replacement with fibrous tissue (to form the ligamentum arteriosum) may not be complete for 4–6 months.

Closure of the ducts venosus remains a mystery. Flow appears to continue for a few hours after birth. There is no clearly defined sphincter between the ductus venosus and the inferior vena cava; nevertheless when placental blood flow ceases the diameter of the opening into the inferior vena cava is reduced and eventually complete closure occurs. In spite of the lack of a defined sphincter or any known chemical stimulus to closure, the ductus venosus is less likely to remain patent than either of the other two shunts. With closure of the shunts the sides of the heart are in series and the adult configuration is now complete.

2.2.3 Changes in cardiac output and blood pressure

Cardiac output is a meaningless term in fetal life because of the shunting of blood. It is almost impossible to measure the direct output of each of the two ventricles. One of the determinants of cardiac output, heart rate, however, is frequently measured. During most of pregnancy the rate is 120–140 beats/min. As far as is known the mechanisms for altering stroke volume are not well developed, so any change in cardiac output is mainly a function of heart rate. Heart rates below 100 and above 180 beats/min are indicative of fetal distress. This is the reason for monitoring heart rate in susceptible individuals during pregnancy. Changes in heart rate are most pronounced during labour. Pressure on the fetal skull may cause an increase in heart rate and bradycardia late in a uterine contraction usually signifies hypoxaemia. The heart rate usually changes during each uterine contraction but should quickly return to normal after the end of the contraction.

After birth, with the normal configuration of the circulation achieved, cardiac output is a more meaningful term signifying the output of each ventricle. In the neonate the normal cardiac output of approximately 180 ml/kg body weight /min is some two- to three-fold that in an adult. As a proportion of body weight this decreases throughout childhood until puberty. Heart rate may rise in the first 1–2 weeks of life but thereafter falls, reaching adult rates at puberty or just after (Fig. 2.4).

Experiments in a number of animals have shown that fetal systolic arterial pressure rises throughout gestation, but even at birth it is relatively low compared to mature animals. In humans, systolic pressure is only 70–80 mmHg (9.3–10.7 kPa) at birth, or as soon after as it can be conveniently measured, but it rises steadily during the first 6 weeks of life and thereafter more slowly until puberty (see Fig. 2.4).

The cardiac sympathetic supply is only partially developed at birth and considerable postnatal development occurs. The increased heart rate after birth is suggested to be a demonstration of the increasing influence of the

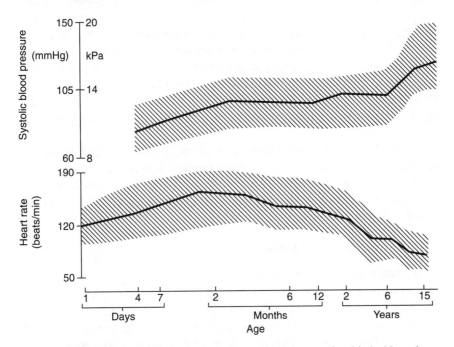

Fig. 2.4. Changes in blood pressure and heart rate after birth. Note the logarithmic scale of the abscissa. Lines indicate mean values and the hatched area is ±2SD. Data taken from Rigby, M.L. and Shinebourne, E.A. (1981). In *Scientific foundations of paediatrics*, 2nd edn, (ed. J.A. Davis, J. Dobbing), Chapter 19. Heinemann, London.

sympathetic system. Parasympathetic supply develops somewhat earlier and reflex control of the heart in the fetus therefore dominates. It is probable that the pronounced fetal bradycardia in response to fetal hypoxaemia depends on parasympathetic reflexes and, hence, it may be prevented or at least reduced by selective parasympathetic blockade. Animal experiments have shown that the fetal heart can respond to sympathetic and parasympathetic neurotransmitters from approximately half way through gestation and baroceptor reflexes are present shortly thereafter. Chemoreceptor reflexes develop at about the same time.

2.2.4 Circulatory problems

The majority of circulatory problems in the neonate arise from two types of problem: congenital malformations, which are outside the scope of this book and asphyxia. Asphyxia after birth can cause a reversal of the changes in the circulation that occur at birth. Pulmonary vessels are very sensitive to hypoxia and constrict, thus raising pulmonary artery pressure and reducing pulmonary blood flow. These changes, if severe enough, increase pulmonary artery pressure until it once again rises above aortic pressure and allows blood to flow through the ductus arteriosus into the aorta—the reduced PO_2 either directly or because of production of mediators such as prostaglandins, allowing relaxation of the muscle of the ductus wall and so allowing it to become patent again. A further consequence is the reduction in left atrial pressure allowing deoxygenated blood from the right atrium to enter through the foramen ovale. This reduces the oxygen delivery to tissues even further and can be fatal. Because of this reversibility the circulation is said to be 'brittle' during the first weeks of life until complete closure of the shunts occurs.

Overloading of the circulation may occur if all the blood from the placenta is drained into the baby before the cord is tied; underloading may result in low blood pressure. These problems usually only occur in premature infants, however, because there is relatively more of the total blood volume present in the placenta (see p. 45).

2.3 The respiratory system

2.3.1 Fetal respiratory movements

Movements of the fetal chest wall analogous to respiratory movements begin very early during gestation although initially they are very irregular. As pregnancy progresses they become more regular and late in pregnancy have been shown to be correlated with fetal EEG waves. Patterns characteristic of rapid eye movement sleep (REM) are associated with rapid (60/min) fetal respiratory movements and in the intervals there are much slower movements or only single movements rather like gasps. Towards term respiratory movements can be seen for up to 90 per cent of the time.

The purpose of these movements is not clear. The fetal lung contains a mixture of amniotic fluid and fluid secreted by the lungs themselves, and chest movements just cause movement of small amounts of fluid into and out of the upper respiratory passages. The movements have no role in gas exchange which is one function of the placenta. The work performed moving the fluid is not strictly isometric, but it may help to increase the force that can be generated by the muscles; considerable force is necessary to enable the baby to take its first breath. Alternatively, the movements may have a role in increasing the capacity of the chest and the size of the lungs prior to birth.

After approximately 24 weeks of gestation, type II pneumocytes begin to secrete surfactant. Secretion rate is greater nearer term, increasing dramatically after 32 weeks and production appears to be under the control of cortisol from the adrenal cortex. 'Surfactant' is a group of closely related phospholipids which lower surface tension at air/liquid interfaces. Because of their unique properties they are able to decrease surface tension (T) in proportion to the thickness of the layer of surfactant. If alveoli become smaller then the surface tension is reduced more. Because the pressure inside a liquid bubble would *increase* as diameter of the bubble decreased if surface tension were constant (according to the law of Laplace, $P = 2T/R$) the presence of surfactant introduces a stabilizing factor, ensuring that small alveoli do not have higher pressures and so empty into larger ones. Of course, surfactant has no role in fetal life since it only acts at air/water interfaces. Adequate amounts are essential for breathing after birth, however, so this is a 'preparatory' function. One use has been made of surfactant by obstetricians. Because it enters amniotic fluid its presence and concentration have been used in diagnostic tests to determine whether a fetus is sufficiently mature to be able to breathe after birth. Such decisions are important for timing planned premature deliveries.

2.3.2 Breathing at birth

At birth there is an abrupt transition from oxygen delivery via the mother and placenta to an air-breathing, independent existence. The first prerequisite is that the lungs be emptied of the fluid they contain, some 30 ml/kg body weight. Much of this is squeezed out by compression of the fetal thorax as it passes through the birth canal. Careful observation will show its exit from the nose or mouth when the head appears during delivery. The remainder is reabsorbed into the pulmonary capillaries and lymphatics. When pulmonary vascular pressure falls the balance of Starling forces in the lung ensures reabsorption of any remaining fluid. Reabsorption is complete within 24–48 h. Babies delivered by Caesarean section do not have the thorax compressed during delivery, but after birth they seem to be able to respire relatively normally, so the reabsorptive mechanisms must be capable of emptying all the fluid from the lungs.

At birth the normal sequence is that the baby gives a deep gasp, which is equivalent to a very deep breath and then gives a cry. Normal respiratory rate is established within minutes. The first breath is normally of 30–40 ml of air and is associated with a very low intrathoracic pressure which may reach 4–10 kPa (40–100 cm H_2O) below atmospheric pressure. It has been suggested that this large negative pressure is necessary to open the lungs initially, rather like blowing up a new balloon. Certainly with the compliance of the lung so low (see Fig. 2.5) large negative pressures are needed.

The problem of why the baby takes its first breath has not been solved. It has been suggested among other reasons that hypoxia, increased sensory stimulation, and even removal of the 'diving' reflex play a role. Hypoxia develops even during a normal delivery and this together with a mild acidosis may help to stimulate the chemoreceptors which begin to function at birth. When the baby is delivered from its sensory-deprived state in the womb to the outside world many sensory stimuli are experienced for the first time and increase neural activity in the reticular formation of the brainstem; it is known from experiments in older children and adults that increased sensory stimulation enhances breathing. The sensory stimuli may

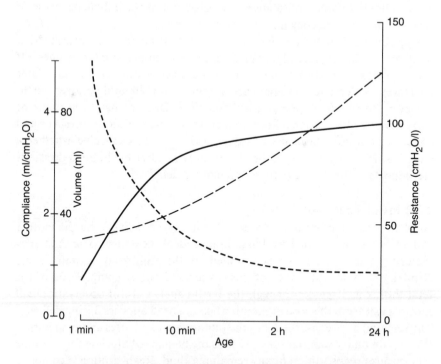

Fig. 2.5. Changes in mechanical properties of the lungs during the first day of life. Note the logarithmic scale of the abscissa. Resting lung volume (——), compliance (– – –), resistance (------). From Godfrey, S. (1981). In *Scientific foundations of paediatrics*, 2nd edn, (ed. J.A. Davis, J. Dobbing), Chapter 21. Heinemann, London.

be increased by a midwife slapping the baby's bottom or sucking mucus from the pharynx and stimulating receptors at the back of the throat. Removal of the face from amniotic fluid may also help to stimulate respiration. In many mammals, but to a lesser extent in adult humans, immersion of the face in water inhibits respiration and if this reflex is present in babies its removal may enhance breathing.

Breathing movements in the fetus are controlled mainly by nervous tissue and the chemoreceptors appear to have little effect until just before delivery. At birth, however, the chemoreceptors, both central and peripheral, become more effective and begin to exercise much more control over respiration. This may be due to an increased blood flow through the chemoreceptors which in turn may be controlled by the sympathetic nervous system.

2.3.3 Respiration after birth

In normal babies breathing becomes regular soon after birth. Within a few minutes the functional residual capacity has increased to 20 ml/kg body weight and this rises over the next few hours to approximately 30 ml/kg. Tidal volume is approximately 20 ml (5–6 ml/kg body weight) and respiratory rate rapid at approximately 30 breaths/min so the total minute ventilation is 500–600 ml/min. The proportion of this which enters the physiological dead space and, thus, is unavailable for gaseous exchange with the capillaries is 30–35 per cent (1.5–2 ml/kg body weight), rather similar to the adult.

Various lung volumes and capacities measured by spirometry are difficult to measure in neonates but it has been possible during periods of crying to measure vital capacity and total lung volume; vital capacity is approximately 30 ml/kg body weight and total lung volume 60 ml/kg. The compliance of the lungs is very small because of the 'stiffness' of the tissues and probably reflects some fluid retention in the interstitial space; compliance rapidly increases over the next few hours. Resistance to air flow falls as lung volume and compliance increase (see Fig. 2.5), so it is obvious that the work of breathing rapidly decreases.

The process of gas transfer in the newborn is thought to be similar to that in adults. It should be remembered, however, that as well as smaller alveoli the newborn only has approximately 10 per cent of the adult number of alveoli and so proportionately makes more use of the respiratory bronchioles. Nor does it have as much carbonic anhydrase, the concentration being 20 per cent of that in adults. This does not seem to impede CO_2 handling however.

2.3.4 Changes in oxygen delivery and usage

Most of the organs of the fetus are supplied by blood with a relatively low O_2 tension (see also Fig. 2.3) and aortic blood has a low saturation. Indeed the hypoxia experienced by the fetus in the uterus has been compared to an adult living on top of Mount Everest. This hypoxia is dramatically changed at birth although PO_2 continues to rise over the next 5 h or so (Fig. 2.6). Thereafter, adult values are almost achieved. Saturation of haemoglobin with oxygen rises from 40–50 per cent in the fetus to 80–90 per cent in the newborn. Changes in PCO_2 are rather slower to occur and are less dramatic overall reflecting the excellent CO_2 exchange that occurs across the placental membranes. PCO_2 may fall below adult levels 2–3 days after birth but over the next week or so values are stabilized at adult levels. The pH of the blood rises much more slowly than the CO_2 falls, probably because the fetus has a metabolic acidosis with elevated blood concentrations of lactate. Even so normal adult pHs are achieved after 1–2 weeks of life (Fig. 2.6).

Oxygen usage by the fetus has not been estimated and even in neonates the measurements are difficult. Since the baby is very sensitive to temperature and when temperature falls dramatically increases its oxygen usage, only oxygen usage measured while the baby is in a thermoneutral environment (see p. 56) is meaningful. Such values are approximately 7 ml oxygen/kg body weight/min which is about twice that of adults. There are similar reasons why it is difficult to measure the respiratory quotient (RQ) but the RQ at birth is thought to be approximately 0.7 and by the end of the first week 0.8.

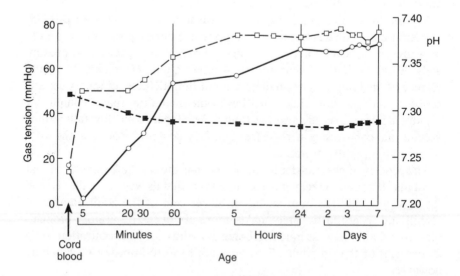

Fig. 2.6. Mean blood gases during the first week of life. Note the logarithmic scale of the abscissa: pH, ○; PO_2, □; PCO_2, ■. From Godfrey, S. (1981). In *Scientific foundations of paediatrics*, 2nd edn, (ed. J.A. Davis, J. Dobbing), Chapter 21. Heinemann, London.

2.3.5 **Pulmonary blood flow**

Pulmonary blood flow in the fetus is very low and most of this blood is shunted from the pulmonary artery through the ductus arteriosus. Effectively then the pressures in the right and left sides of the heart are similar and this is reflected in the relatively equal thicknesses of the right and left ventricular walls. The lung arterioles are constricted because they are exquisitely sensitive to PO_2 and the PO_2 in the fluid filling the lungs is low. This also helps to raise the pressure in the pulmonary circulation. The muscular walls of the pulmonary arterioles and even the pulmonary arteries are thicker than in adults; the wall thickness:diameter ratio is very high when compared to adults. After the baby takes its first breath, however, the arterioles dilate due to the increase in PO_2 in alveolar air and over the next 4 months or so there is an increasing dilatation of the pulmonary arterial vessels. Muscular development lags behind until the adult ratio of thickness:diameter is achieved at 4–6 months of age. Thereafter, muscular development of the walls proceeds *pari passu* with the increase in diameter.

2.3.6 **Problems with breathing**

The major problems with breathing at birth are due to obstruction of the airway, asphyxia during birth, or lack of surfactant. Mechanical obstruction of the airways by mucus can give rise to problems but respiratory movements are present (at least initially) and the diagnosis and cure should be obvious.

Asphyxia can give rise to greater problems. Compression of the umbilical cord during delivery, early placental separation from the uterus before the baby is fully delivered, and even prolonged labour can exacerbate the normal hypoxia that occurs during delivery and the normal pattern of breathing may be changed. Basically the hypoxia depresses neural control mechanisms and, subsequently, respiration movements are weaker than normal. The massive effort required to take the first breath may never be achieved. If the mother has received sedatives which are respiratory depressants during labour (for example, pethidine) then the condition will be made much worse. After the initial gasp, if indeed there is one, the baby becomes apnoeic—this is primary apnoea. During this period stimulation of respiration by any means will produce a series of gasps but these may not be forceful enough to delivery oxygen into the lungs.

If any of the gasps result in the baby taking a breath and air enters the lungs, then the period of apnoea terminates. If this is not the case the response to respiratory stimuli gets weaker and weaker, respiratory movements eventually cease, and the baby goes into secondary or terminal apnoea. Positive pressure respiration, forcing oxygen into the lungs, may get round the problem. Premature infants also have problems even after the first breath has been taken, probably because the neural mechanisms for maintaining breathing are not fully developed and they may be subject to periods of apnoea after birth. It has been suggested that this could be a contributing cause to sudden infant death syndrome (SIDS) or cot death but whether this is so is not certain. Recent evidence suggests that letting babies sleep on their backs, not on their tummies, not overheating the room for the baby (that is, allowing increased thermal stimuli, increased metabolism, and, hence, increased CO_2 to help drive respiration) and preventing passive smoking by stopping the parents smoking in the house can reduce the incidence of SIDS by up to 50 per cent. The significance of a recent report that retarded development of the kidneys contributes is not yet clear.

Apnoea may also occur during feeding in the early neonatal period. If it does it is followed by a period of cyanosis. While it is very rare in breast-fed babies it may occur in up to 50 per cent of those fed by bottle. The remedy is simple; remove the bottle and encourage the baby to belch, a process known colloquially as 'winding'.

Lack of surfactant causes respiratory distress syndrome (previously called hyaline membrane disease after the appearance at post-mortem when the alveoli are filled with amorphous, eosinophilic-staining material). Lack of surfactant occurs predominantly in premature babies, before sufficient is produced or in babies born to diabetic or pre-diabetic mothers where the reduced cortisol levels result in lower production of surfactant. The surface tension of the alveoli is unusually high and the mechanical effort required to expand the lungs is excessive. Collapse of the alveoli occurs at the end of a breath and so each breath becomes an exaggerated 'first' breath. Usually, the intrapleural pressures generated are so large that the intercostal muscles cannot resist the inward suction and are drawn inwards. The extra work of breathing requires extra energy and, hence, extra oxygen and the net result is that the baby cannot obtain sufficient oxygen, becomes cyanosed, and is gasping for breath. Sprays containing surfactant have been used to try and alleviate the condition but the results are, in general, disappointing; cortico-steroids have been given to stimulate production of surfactant but in general the treatment is directed towards supplying sufficient oxygen to the neonate (either by artificial ventilation or by an incubator, see p. 59) until the pneomocytes have produced enough of their own surfactant to ameliorate the condition.

2.4 Blood and body fluids

2.4.1 Body fluids

The fetus contains relatively more water than adults or neonates. In early embryos it may account for over 90 per cent of body weight and even though this decreases towards term it is still 80 per cent compared with the

72 per cent of lean body mass in adults. Much of the extra water is extracellular and throughout fetal life the volume of extracellular fluid exceeds that of intracellular fluid.

There are no dramatic changes in body fluid volume at the moment of birth except in blood (see below) but over the next few days there is a decrease in total body water—the loss being almost totally at the expense of the extracellular compartment—and within 2 months after birth body fluid volumes are proportionally the same as those seen in adults. Since the amount of fat in babies is relatively small the percentage of total body water approaches 72 per cent more closely than in the adult.

Fluid balance in the neonate can be a problem. The baby has little control over its fluid intake. Most fluid is given at feeding time as milk and between feeds the baby cannot easily communicate a feeling of thirst. Fluid losses are necessarily high because of increased insensible water loss from the skin (the surface area:volume ratio is high), from the respiratory tract (the respiratory rate is high) and via faeces.

Because of the neonate's small size the loss of fluid has much more serious consequences than in an adult and since the kidney cannot concentrate urine well (see p. 63) there is always the chance of dehydration.

2.4.2 Blood

While changes in blood volume in general follow the changes in extracellular fluid there are important changes around birth. At any one time, approximately 35 per cent of the circulating blood in the fetus is present in the placenta. When the placenta is delivered after the baby, the attending midwife or obstetrician ties the umbilical cord cutting off a certain amount of blood in the placenta. Practices vary but some would tie the cord early, depriving the baby of some of the placental blood while others, by delaying tying the cord and sometimes by raising the placenta above the baby, effectively give the baby a blood transfusion. The benefits of this placental transfusion are not clear. Certainly the kidney rapidly excretes the extra fluid component, but the red cells are retained (see below).

2.4.3 Blood cells

2.4.3.1 *Red blood cells*

Red blood cells are produced in different organs at different stages of development. The first red cells are produced 5–6 weeks after conception within blood vessels in the yolk sac, but shortly thereafter extravascular manufacture begins in the liver. From 3 to 6 months of intrauterine life the red cells are produced predominantly in the liver although during that time the spleen produces an increasing fraction and the bone marrow begins to produce erythrocytes. During the last 3 months of gestation production of red cells declines in the liver, peaks then declines in the spleen and increases gradually in the marrow until at birth most red blood cells are produced in the marrow. Initially all the bone marrow is concerned but throughout childhood the fraction of marrow producing red cells gradually declines until in the adult only the marrow of flat bones, the skull, and vertebrae are involved.

The numbers of red cells increase dramatically throughout gestation from $1-1.5 \times 10^{12}/l$ at 10 weeks to adult numbers $4.5-5 \times 10^{12}/l$ at birth, and because of the increased production 3–5 per cent are reticulocytes with frequent nucleated red cells. The size of the red cells reduces dramatically over that period and from initially very large cells at 10 weeks (MCV $\cong 220$ fl) the cells decline until they reach approximately 110 fl at birth. The cells are still markedly larger than adult cells, however. The amount of haemoglobin also increases during gestation from 6–6.5 g/dl (3.5–3.9 mmol/l of the monomer) to levels exceeding those of adults 16–17 g/dl (9.5–10.1 mmoles/l). For some reason not yet fully understood the fragility of red cells in the

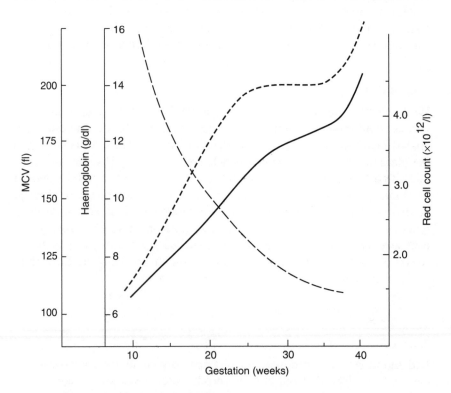

Fig. 2.7. Haemoglobin concentration (-----), red cell count (——), and mean red cell volume (MCV, ---) in the human fetus. Data from Black, P.J. and Berkham, P. (1981). In *Scientific foundations of paediatrics*, 2nd edn, (ed. J.A. Davis, J. Dobbing), Chapter 25. Heinemann, London.

fetus is greater than that of adult cells and their mean life expectancy is reduced from 120 to approximately 60 days. Whether this reflects differences in pH in the fetal blood, different membrane proteins, or an influence of fetal haemoglobin is uncertain. After birth there is rapid breakdown of a number of red cells and because the liver is immature and not able to cope with the bilirubin formed as a consequence of this breakdown, neonates frequently became jaundiced. Because the bilirubin is not conjugated and hence is lipid soluble, it may cross the immature blood–brain barrier and be deposited in brain tissues—especially the basal ganglia and if in excess cause damage—a condition known as kernicterus.

2.4.3.2 *Haemoglobin*

The haemoglobin concentration and haematocrit rise rapidly during the first hours after birth probably due to excretion of fluid and this occurs whether or not there is marked placental transfusion. After a few days there is a gradual fall in haemoglobin concentration until levels lower than those found in adults are the norm, regardless again of whether or not there was a placental transfusion (Fig. 2.8). Even at 2 years of age the child may still on average have a low haemoglobin concentration but by puberty the concentration has crept up to adult values.

The type of haemoglobin present in the fetus is different from the adult. While the adult (HbA) has a tetrameric molecule with 2α- and 2β-chains of globin, in the fetus the 2β-chains are substituted by 2γ-chains (HbF). There are six possible variants of the haemoglobin chain $\alpha,\beta,\gamma,\delta,\zeta$ and ϵ. As can be seen (Fig. 2.9) ζ and ϵ are embryonic forms which disappear by about the third month of life as the proportion of α-chain increases; δ is present only in very small amounts. The major changes around birth take place in β and γ. Around the sixth to seventh month of intrauterine life the fetus begins to produce β-chains and by birth somewhere between 50 and 75 per cent of cells contain only HbA. Thereafter only α- and β-chains are produced.

The functional significance of the presence of HbF lies in its greater affinity than HbA for oxygen presumably because it is not affected by 2-3DPG. In comparable oxygen tensions fetal Hb will saturate to a greater extent than HbA so that even though the partial pressures of oxygen are very similar in mother and fetus more oxygen will be carried by the HbF. This enables the fetus to survive at a PO_2 which has been compared to that of an adult at the summit of Mount Everest. One of the unanswered questions in fetal physiology is what the stimulus is to change from HbF to HbA production.

Overall control of red cell production is similar to that in the adult. Erythropoietin is produced by fetal liver and kidney. Because of the low PO_2 in the fetus the concentration of erythropoietin is very high. After birth however, the sudden rise in PO_2 results in a fall of erythropoietin to unmeasurable levels. This contributes to the first part of the physiological anaemia. Over the succeeding months the concentration of PO_2 at which erythropoietin is stimulated, increases, until eventually it settles at adult values.

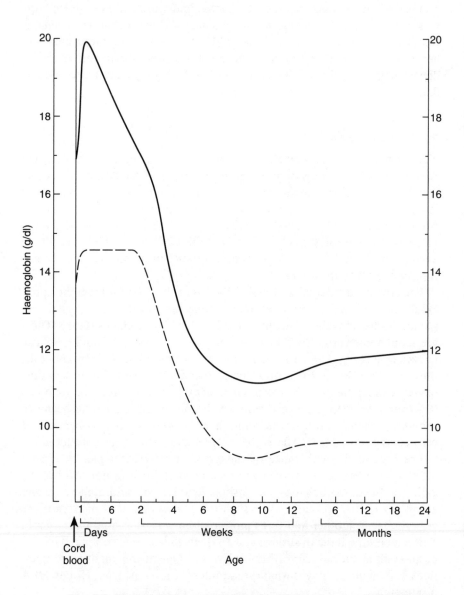

Fig. 2.8. Haemoglobin concentration in the first 2 years of life showing mean value (——) and lower limit of normality (---). Data from Black, P.J. and Berkham, P. (1981). In *Scientific foundations of paediatrics*, 2nd edn, (ed. J.A. Davis, J. Dobbing), Chapter 25. Heinemann, London.

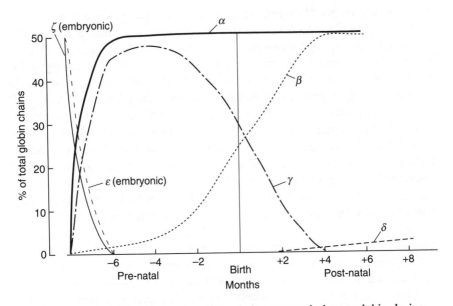

Fig. 2.9. The changes in globin chains present in haemoglobin during fetal and neonatal life.

2.4.3 *White cells*

Less is known about white cell production in the fetus. It begins at approximately the same time as erythropoiesis but occurs mainly in the bone marrow, spleen, and lymph nodes although early development does also involve the liver. At about the twentieth week of gestation the granulocytes are approximately $1 \times 10^9/l$ and lymphocytes $4 \times 10^9/l$. By term the granulocyte concentration has increased to $8 \times 10^9/l$ but lymphocytes remain the same. The granulocyte count increases for 24 h after birth but then falls back to adult levels during days 4–7. Lymphocyte numbers increase after birth and reach a maximum at approximately 6 months of age when they exceed granulocyte numbers at $7.5 \times 10^9/l$. After the first year of life these then decline until they reach adult numbers by about 16 years. Thus, for a period in childhood lymphocytes are the predominant white blood cells.

Much is being learned about factors such as growth colony stimulating factors (GCSF) which can stimulate white cell growth. The role they play in the fetus and the neonate is not yet resolved however.

2.5 The gastrointestinal tract and metabolism

2.5.1 Gastrointestinal function in the fetus

The fetus obtains all its nutritional requirements from the mother via the placenta (see Chapter 1). Glucose, which supplies most of the energy, amino acids, which are used for protein synthesis and gluconeogensis, and fatty acids cross the placenta easily but the passage of some lipids is restricted.

Plasma glucose concentration in the fetus is approximately 3 mmol/l, almost half that of adults but its control is poor. Insulin and glucagon do not exert their normal level of control and while disastrously low levels are prevented by the autonomic nervous system and adrenalin, fetal levels tend to reflect maternal levels. This is especially so in fetuses of diabetic mothers where the high maternal blood glucose is reflected in a higher than normal fetal blood glucose, in spite of a higher than usual fetal insulin concentration. Fetal plasma concentration of amino acids is much higher than maternal but this probably reflects the active transport mechanisms of the placenta rather than metabolism of the fetus. Towards the end of gestation, relatively large amounts of glycogen are stored in fetal muscle and liver, and fat stores, both brown and white, are laid down. This stored energy is necessary for the newborn baby's survival before feeding is initiated.

Swallowing is established early in fetal life and amniotic fluid enters the stomach. Most other gut movements are rudimentary, however and colonic movements are minimal. Meconium (see p. 51) which is present in the gut before term is not usually found in amniotic fluid. It may be that this lack of movement reflects the very low levels of motilin (see p. 52).

Secretion by salivary glands and amylase production occurs in the second half of pregnancy and it appears that pancreatic secretion occurs at approximately the same time. At the fourth to fifth month of gestation gastric glands begin to appear but do not seem to secrete since gastric contents at birth are neutral.

2.5.2 Changes in gastrointestinal function at birth

At birth the intravenous nutrition of the fetus ceases but oral feeding does not begin for several hours or days. Over this time the neonate depends on the metabolic stores laid down late in gestation; premature babies obviously have a problem because of reduced stores.

Blood glucose concentration increases during parturition probably as a result of the high concentrations of circulating catecholamines and increased activity of the sympathetic nervous system causing glycogenolysis.

2.5.3 Changes in gastrointestinal function in the neonate

There is still considerable debate about the optimum time to give the newborn baby its first feed. Custom, hospital routine, convenience, social factors, and much mythology seem to play at least as large a part as physiology in this decision. Feeding has a profound effect on the gastrointestinal tract. Growth of the GI tract is very rapid but only if food enters the lumen. If watery solutions are given or the baby is fasted no growth occurs, but if milk is fed the gut doubles in size within approximately 24 h. This may be due to the nutritional components, although high concentrations of growth factors such as epithelial growth factor (EGF) or insulin-like growth factor (IGF) in the colostrum or milk have also been implicated. In addition, of course, relatively large volumes of milk need to be mixed, propelled, digested, and absorbed efficiently. Since babies born even up to 2 months prematurely also rapidly adapt to feeding it is suggested that there is an environmental trigger to the changes that occur.

When neonatal feeding is established the major energy source changes from glucose, in the fetus, to fats which are present in human milk at high concentrations. So, with new sources of energy the infant has to maintain metabolic homeostasis unaided. Most of the consequent changes depend on gastrointestinal hormones.

2.5.4 Digestion and absorption

The mechanisms responsible for digestion and absorption are the same in neonates as in adults with two notable exceptions. Lactose is the major carbohydrate in milk and this is usually hydrolysed by a specific disaccharidase, lactase, in the brush border of the small intestine. The amounts of the different disaccharidases present are determined by the diet (that is they are inducible) so the amount of lactase is much higher than in adults.

Absorption of specific proteins is also different. Breast-fed babies have raised concentrations of plasma immunoglobulin (particularly IgA, IgG, and IgM) when compared with bottle-fed babies. These large molecules probably cross the intestinal wall by pinocytosis. The length of time that this mechanism exists in neonatal life varies from species to species. In humans it is not known how long it persists—certainly a matter of months. Such transfer of immunoglobulin accounts for the passive transfer of immunity from mother to child which is a feature of early life.

2.5.5 Gastrointestinal motility

This has not been studied extensively. The first stool is usually passed on the first day of life and consists of a sticky black or dark green mass called meconium. It consists of epithelial cells, intestinal secretions, bile pigments, and large amounts of proteoglycans which are the undigested residues of the mucus secretion from all parts of the gut. Meconium usually disappears in 2–3 days to be replaced by a green–brown greasy stool which contains a large amount of fat, a result of incomplete lipid digestion due to immature pancreatic secretion. This gradually changes to the yellow semi-liquid stool of the breast-fed baby. Cow's milk makes the stools much firmer even if it is introduced into the diet in only small amounts. Bowel motions are much more frequent in the neonate than the adult. This can cause a lot of parental distress. There is great variability, however and while there may be up to 12 stools a day, even a normal baby may go 4–5 days without a motion. Defecation is reflex and full control is not gained until the second or third year of life.

2.5.6 Changes in gastrointestinal hormones

Many of the gastrointestinal hormones are secreted during fetal life. There is evidence from animal studies that enteroglucagon, gastrin, glucose-dependent insulin-releasing peptide (GIP), pancreatic polypeptide, and bombesin are secreted and these have also been detected in amniotic fluid in humans. Gastrin concentration (in human fetuses) is low at 20 weeks of gestation when compared with adults but rises thereafter. Any fetal results must be treated cautiously, however, since concentrations of all the hormones vary with the condition of the fetus. Perhaps most noteworthy in this respect is motilin the concentration of which is increased in fetal distress; this increase probably accounts for the increased intestinal motility which causes meconium to be passed into the amniotic fluid in this condition. Meconium-stained amniotic fluid has long been recognized as a sign of fetal distress.

Motilin, GIP, gastrin, enteroglucagon, and pancreatic polypeptide all increase immediately after the first feed and achieve plasma concentrations much greater than those in the adult (Fig. 2.10). If oral feeding is delayed so are the changes in gastrointestinal hormones. Peak basal (that is between meals) plasma concentrations of the peptides are reached in the first or second week of extrauterine life. The normal hormonal response to a meal takes rather longer to develop and it may be 2–4 months before the adult pattern of response to a meal is established. There appears to be a neurally mediated reflex which stimulates both gastrointestinal and pancreatic hormones in response to a meal with potentiation of the pancreatic hormone secretion by GIP, although enteroglucagon, bombesin, cholecystokinin-pancreozymin (CCK-PZ), and neurotensin may all play a role.

The reason for the persistently raised basal concentrations is not clear. Relative to enterocytes the endocrine cell mass in the neonatal gut is much greater than in the adult and the gut peptides may have a special role to play in the postnatal mechanisms of the gastrointestinal tract. However, a contributing factor to the increase in gut peptides may be a deficiency of the mechanism which normally removes the peptides from plasma. Most of the hormones have been discovered to cause growth, at least in adults and it may be they have a special role to play in the very rapid growth of the gut. Gastrin and enteroglucagon, in addition to other actions, stimulate growth of gut mucosa. Gastrin, CCK-PZ, and pancreatic polypeptide may stimulate growth of the endocrine pancreas, while motilin increases motility of the

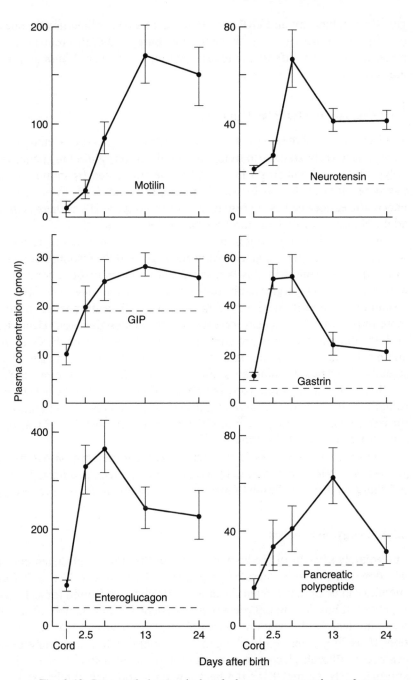

Fig. 2.10. Postnatal changes in basal plasma concentrations of gastro-intestinal hormones. Each neonate gave only one datum point. Broken lines show mean adult fasting values. From Lucas, A. (1981). In *Scientific foundations of paediatrics*, 2nd edn, (ed. J.A. Davis, J. Dobbing), Chapter 6. Heinemann, London.

gut. Enteroglucagon and GIP are major factors controlling insulin release (see below). Whether these changes contribute to the different hormone patterns seen when infants are breast- or bottle-fed (even if human milk is used) remains to be discovered.

2.5.7 Changes in insulin and glucagon

The Islets of Langerhans contain the four principal cell types seen in adults from a very early stage of development and insulin, glucagon, pancreatic polypeptide, and somatostatin can all be demonstrated by immunofluorescent techniques. By birth there is probably about four times as much pancreatic endocrine tissue present relative to body weight as there is in the adult. Neonates of diabetic mothers may have even more.

Neither insulin nor glucagon, however, seem to be associated pre-natally with regulation of plasma glucose concentration and the response of insulin to a hyperglycaemic stimulus is delayed and appears to be related to the duration of the hyperglycaemia rather than its magnitude. The effect of insulin on promoting amino acid transfer across cell membranes seems to be more important. Amino acid increase also stimulates glucagon release and both insulin and glucagon are stimulated by adrenergic stimuli. Glucagon and insulin may act together to stimulate growth. However, in view of the recently described insulin-like growth factors (IGF), it is now unclear whether earlier results, reporting the effects of insulin, could have been due to IGF. At birth there is a surge of glucagon secretion and this alteration of the insulin:glucagon ratio may be one reason for mobilization of free fatty acids which occurs at this time.

After the first few weeks of extrauterine life the insulin response to hyperglycaemia develops and eventually assumes the role seen in adults. There is still a large reflex stimulation of insulin and glucagon in response to feeding.

2.5.8 Energy metabolism

Immediately after birth the baby depends on the store of glycogen and fat laid down in the later stages of pregnancy. These have to last until fresh supplies can be obtained from the milk. Liver glycogen is used for as long as supplies last but the amount present at birth depends on a number of factors including length of gestation, placental insufficiency, and maternal nutrition. If feeding is delayed too long in the neonate profound hypoglycaemia can occur. Plasma glucose is normally raised at birth (see p. 50), falls to approximately 3 mmol/l for the next few days and then climbs gradually until adult concentrations are reached between 1 and 6 months.

From approximately 2 h after birth the free fatty acid concentration in the plasma rises rapidly. A slow decline then occurs until adult concentrations are reached at approximately 1 year. Interestingly, exposure to cold causes hydrolysis of brown adipose tissue (see p. 57) whereas 'starvation' results in hydrolysis of white fat. Fat supply in the milk is important in maintaining plasma glucose. Even supplying gluconeogenic amino acids will not maintain blood glucose in the absence of fats. The oxidation of fats is necessary to sustain a high rate of gluconeogenesis.

2.5.9 Liver function

Many of the liver's functions are similar to the adult although less well developed. However, in fetal life glycogen deposition depends on the provision of substrates such as lactate and glucose is not converted to glycogen in any significant amount. Even before birth the liver has significant amounts of galactokinase, an enzyme which converts galactose to glucose and, thence, into glycogen. Lack of galactose pre-natally prevents the enzyme being useful at this time. Glucose is not converted to glycogen directly even in the neonate, but galactose uptake (derived from lactose in the milk) results in galactose uptake to the liver. In the presence of insulin this induces production of glycogen synthetase and, thus, deposition of glycogen.

Other enzyme systems may be absent or present in only small amounts. For example, the enzymes necessary for conjugation of bilirubin are low at birth but increase rapidly. This immaturity, combined with the increased breakdown of blood derived from the placenta (see p. 47) results in a physiological jaundice in the first few days of life. Related aspects of detoxification are also immature and so many drugs or hormones have a prolonged half-life. Drugs should be used cautiously in neonates.

2.5.10 Gastrointestinal problems

There are several different classes of problem that can affect the neonatal gastrointestinal tract. One major problem is caused by lack of specific digestive enzymes, such as lactase or a generalized reduction or lack of enzymes from the pancreas in diseases such as cystic fibrosis. The resultant reduction of digestion and absorption causes diarrhoea of varying degrees of severity.

Vomiting and diarrhoea cause problems to the neonate, whatever the primary cause, because of the loss of water and electrolytes. Diarrhoea may be associated with infection or disturbed digestive (lactase deficiency) or absorptive (such as the rare congenital chloride diarrhoea) function. Vomiting can be spectacular if due to pyloric stenosis or other mechanical obstruction of the tract, but even normal babies usually regurgitate some food after a feed, especially if they are not 'winded' properly: this probably occurs because the lower oesophageal sphincter is not fully competent.

Hypoglycaemia can arise from a variety of causes. The signs are relatively non-specific and range from enhanced activity (such as twitching, occasional convulsions, or a high pitched crying) to reduced activity (limpness, difficulty in feeding, or coma). The neonatal nervous system, however, appears much more tolerant of hypoglycaemia than its adult counterpart. Neonatal neural tissue can use metabolic substrates other than glucose quite efficiently.

2.6 Temperature regulation

Closely related to metabolic regulation is temperature regulation and it is sensible to consider it at this point.

2.6.1 The thermoneutral zone after birth

The fetus has no problems with temperature regulation since it is surrounded by amniotic fluid at body temperature, which acts as a heat sink. The mother assumes responsibility for supplying or dissipating heat. At birth there are dramatic changes in environmental temperature as the neonate is pushed into a cold cruel world. The change is reduced by keeping modern obstetrical units at a high temperature—but this is still some 8–10°C below the temperature of amniotic fluid.

The newborn baby is homoeothermic and defends its body temperature by a series of mechanisms for altering heat loss and heat production. While these mechanisms have parallels in adults their relative importance is different in the neonate.

The thermoneutral zone (see Chapter 6) is defined as the range of environmental temperature over which metabolic rate is kept at a minimum. Within this zone, temperature regulation is achieved by changes in skin blood flow. The zone is much higher in a naked neonate (32–36°C) than in a naked adult (27–31°C). It must be remembered that clothing provides a microclimate around the body which helps to achieve this temperature.

2.6.2 Special problems of the neonate

The major problem of the neonate in maintaining body temperature is to retain body heat. The surface area to volume ratio is high as in any small mammal and, since loss of heat is dependent on surface area while generation of heat (that is, metabolic rate) depends on body mass or volume, anything which increases the ratio causes problems with retention of sufficient heat to maintain temperature. The neonate has additional problems. Immediately after birth the baby is wet and evaporation of amniotic fluid can cause loss of a tremendous amount of heat. Neonates have only a thin layer of subcutaneous fat to help insulate the skin. The size of the head in a baby is disproportionate to the body size and has a copious blood supply. It therefore represents a potential large heat loss. Clothing, especially woolly bonnets, can help to decrease this heat loss.

All the above problems are magnified in small infants whether preterm or small for dates. In general the smaller the baby, the greater the problem.

2.6.3 Heat production

There are only limited means at the disposal of a neonate to combat loss of heat. Voluntary muscular activity and behavioural responses which are common in adults (see Chapter 6) are not viable options. Shivering which also occurs in adults does not occur in neonates. Whether this is because the appropriate neuromuscular apparatus for shivering is not sufficiently developed in neonates or whether the threshold temperature at which shivering would occur is so low that other mechanisms supervene is not known. Metabolic activity in all cells, but especially in the liver, heart, and brain produces a fixed amount of heat. As the baby grows metabolic rate increases, for example, oxygen usage, a useful measure of energy production, doubles in the first 10 days of life.

Probably the major generator of extra heat to combat heat loss is brown adipose tissue. Brown adipose tissue (BAT) is a specialized energy source. In contrast to ordinary white adipose tissue it has a good blood supply, a well developed sympathetic nerve supply, and many mitochondria surrounding numerous small vacuoles filled with fat. When the vacuoles are full of fat the tissue is yellow, but as the vacuoles empty the tissue takes on a brown coloration (hence, its name), because of the high content of mitochondrial cytochrome enzymes. Energy is produced by the breakdown of the lipids. Whereas in white adipose tissue lipolysis occurs and the products, glycerol and fatty acids, are transported to other sites, the mitochondria in BAT are able to utilize the fatty acids themselves, eventually deriving energy from the tricarboxylic acid cycle. Fatty acids or a derivative have a second effect in BAT. They increase production of a 32 kDa uncoupling protein. Normally mitochondria generate a significant proton gradient across their membranes, but the uncoupling protein acts as a channel which dissipates the gradient so that although the tricarboxylic acid cycle keeps turning the energy generated is dissipated and not converted to ATP. This of course generates much local heat.

In human neonates BAT is present in a thin sheet between the scapulae, around the neck, behind the sternum, and around the kidneys and adrenals (Fig. 2.11). The amount and location is very variable in different species. In a normal newborn baby BAT accounts for 2–6 per cent of the total body weight. Once the stores have been depleted the baby has few defences against cold. Although BAT is present from the fifth month of gestation most of it is laid down during the last weeks before birth and premature infants, who need it most, have reduced amounts. Some BAT persists to adolescence but its major function is during the first 6 months of life. The function and amount in adults is debatable.

The response of the neonate to cold is integrated in the hypothalamus and mediated mainly through the sympathetic nerve supply to BAT. The sympathetic nerve terminals release noradrenalin which acts on a unique β_3-receptor to stimulate thermogenesis. The whole process can be controlled at a cellular level to deliver variable amounts of heat, but the details are not yet known.

2.6.4 Heat loss

Mechanisms to increase heat loss in the neonate are not well developed. In the UK this is not a problem, except perhaps in closed cars exposed to direct sunlight on a hot day. If a baby has to lose excess heat and there is a high

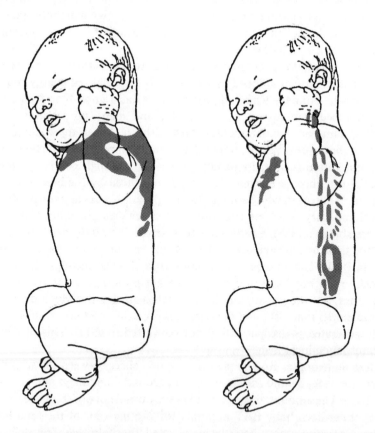

Fig. 2.11. Location of brown adipose tissue (shaded areas) in the human neonate. From Dawkins, M.J.R. and Hull, D. (1965). The production of fat. *Scientific American*, **213**, 63. Copyright © 1965, by Scientific American, Inc. All rights reserved.

environmental temperature, vasodilation is of little help because when environmental temperature exceeds body temperature vasodilation will *increase* the heat delivered to the body. Only evaporation of sweat can therefore be effective, but sweating is not well developed in infants. Sweat glands are present but the increase in body temperature necessary to stimulate sweating is much greater in neonates than in adults. The number of active sweat glands reaches a maximum at approximately 2 years of age but many glands even though appearing anatomically normal do not secrete even in adult life.

Heat loss can be minimized by reducing blood flow to the skin and this is controlled by the autonomic nervous system. Because the autonomic nervous system is not fully developed the baby is not as capable as the adult of dealing with small temperature changes and, hence, the higher thermo-neutral zone.

2.6.5 Consequences of different mechanisms

In spite of the potential problems, most babies have little difficulty in regulating their body temperature. By providing adequate clothing, particularly for the head, hands, and feet and a reasonably warm environment parents can ensure that undue amounts of BAT are not used under 'normal' conditions.

For some babies, however, it is necessary to monitor their temperature more closely. Premature babies have increased problems with temperature regulation and may not be able to manage unaided. Ill babies also have increased problems because the supply of nutrients is reduced and because, for a variety of clinical reasons, it is necessary to nurse them either naked or with minimal clothing. In these conditions it is far easier to maintain the temperature in a closely regulated environment.

2.6.6 Use of incubators

When babies are having difficulty in maintaining body temperature or if they are likely to have such difficulties, then it is convenient to nurse them in a closed environment where the temperature of the air can be raised. The design of incubators is such that air flows over the baby and that there is sufficient movement to mix the air adequately and maintain a stable temperature. The air movement brings its own problems since it results in a large loss of water from exposed skin and this can compromise the fluid balance. Because of this, the humidity of the air also has to be controlled. The precise temperature in the incubator needs to be optimally set for each individual and body temperature must be continuously monitored. Care must also be taken to avoid excessive radiant heat through the perspex canopy which can greatly increase the temperature inside the incubator; as discussed above the neonate has inadequate mechanisms to deal with such a heat load.

As well as controlling temperature incubators can also be used to change the atmosphere around the neonate. If a baby has respiratory difficulties it may be advantageous to increase the ambient pressure of oxygen. Originally 100 per cent oxygen was used to do this but it was shown that long-term this caused fibrosis behind the lens of the eye (retrolental fibroplasia) which ultimately leads to blindness. In the short-term 100 per cent O_2 may also interfere with surfactant production which is a further disadvantage. Partial pressure of oxygen is usually kept below 300 mmHg (40 kPa) and even this pressure can be maintained for only short lengths of time. Since most incubators use a flow-through system (as opposed to a recycling system) which vents to the air there is no build up of carbon dioxide.

2.7 Renal function and fluid balance

2.7.1 Renal function in the fetus

As discussed above the fetus has a higher water content than the adult (see p. 44) and during fetal life the major organ of homeostasis is the placenta. Throughout this time, however, the kidneys are growing and maturing. Those glomeruli deepest in the kidney (the juxtamedullary ones) mature first and not all the cortical glomeruli function at birth. Even allowing for the smaller size of the fetus, renal blood flow is less than in the newborn partly because of incomplete glomerular development and partly due to arteriolar vasoconstriction. A lower glomerular filtration rate (GFR), occurs *pari passu* with the lower blood flow.

In spite of the reduced glomerular filtration, copious amounts of urine are produced by the fetus. This is because the fractional excretion of sodium (that is, the fraction of the sodium filtered at the glomerulus which is not reabsorbed by the nephron) is very high; at 4 months gestation 13 per cent is not reabsorbed, while at term approximately 3.5 per cent is not absorbed compared with 0.3–0.5 per cent in an adult. As sodium is not reabsorbed water is also excreted. Urine flow in the fetus can be monitored using ultrasonic techniques. From these scans it is possible to 'see' the bladder fill and empty regularly. The excreted urine contributes the major fraction to the amniotic fluid; if the kidneys are congenitally absent there is a great reduction in amniotic fluid (oligohydramnios) and this restricts mobility of the fetal limbs, frequently resulting in deformation of limbs or even ears. The failure of the kidney to reabsorb more of the filtered sodium has yet to be explained; immaturity of the reabsorption mechanism or the presence of a specific inhibitor of sodium reabsorption have both been suggested.

Early in gestation it has been shown that the urine produced by the fetal kidney is isotonic. As pregnancy proceeds, however, the urine becomes hypotonic and as a result amniotic fluid is hypotonic. Studies in animals have shown that, at least towards the end of pregnancy, the renal medulla is hypertonic to plasma so although the 'machinery' is in place to produce a concentrated urine the kidney does not do so. Presumably there is insufficient circulating antidiuretic hormone to increase the permeability of distal parts of the nephron but whether this is due to reduced secretion or lack of receptor activity is not known. Because amniotic fluid is hypotonic an osmotic gradient exists with the maternal tissues and considerable loss of fluid occurs across the chorioallantoic membranes. This balances the fluid produced by the kidneys.

2.7.2 Renal changes at birth

Before birth the kidneys can excrete extravagant amounts of salt and water with impunity as any deficiencies are corrected by the placenta. Once the umbilical cord is cut fluid losses must balance fluid intake. While the changes in renal function are not as spectacularly rapid as those in the cardiorespiratory system they are no less significant. Here the changes occur over a few days rather than minutes.

For the first few hours after birth renal function, with respect to GFR and fractional sodium excretion, is similar to the immediate pre-natal levels. Over the next 24–48 h both fall rapidly and then in the succeeding week gradually recover as the baby takes in more fluid. The size of the placental transfusion (see p. 45) determines to some extent the magnitude of the natriuresis and diuresis which occurs during the first few hours. Certainly for the first few hours the baby goes into negative fluid balance and the major loss is borne by the extracellular fluid compartment, which shrinks until it is less than the intracellular fluid compartment. Balance occurs after 7–10 days of life when urine production and GFR increase.

Plasma urea concentration decreases consistently over the first week of life as does plasma creatinine concentration. Since GFR is proportional to the inverse of the plasma creatinine this fall is due to the increasing GFR which occurs after the first 24–48 h. The decrease in plasma urea is more difficult to explain. It may be that for urea the kidney is a more efficient excreting organ than the placenta or that some of the urea in the fetus was transferred across the placenta from the mother.

2.7.3 Renal function in the neonate

It is clear that the neonatal kidney is far from mature in many respects. Both GFR and tubular function are proportionately less than in the adult and remain so until the second year of life.

Glomerular filtration rate rises rapidly from 2–3 days after birth to achieve adult rates (when related to body surface area) after 2–3 years of life (Fig. 2.12). There are a number of reasons for this increase. First, the cortical glomeruli mature; these were non-functional at birth. Secondly, there is an increase in the filtration permeability of the glomerulus which may double in the first year of life. Thirdly, there is an increase in cardiac output (see p. 37) and this increases blood flow to the kidneys. Fourthly, the proportion of this increased cardiac output which goes to the kidneys, increases rapidly; this occurs because the vascular resistance of the kidney decreases more rapidly than any other vascular bed except the lungs. Both these latter changes increase renal blood flow and since renal plasma flow is a major determinant of GFR there is a consequent increase in GFR. In addition, the decreased vascular resistance which is mainly due to relaxation of the afferent arterioles results in an increased pressure in the glomerular capillaries and, hence, a greater mean ultrafiltration pressure. Direct measurements in guinea-pigs have shown that the effective ultrafiltration pressure rises two- or three-fold in early post-natal life. Because the outer cortical glomeruli become functional, progressively more blood goes to the outer parts of the renal cortex than in the fetus.

It is not possible to generalize about the development of tubular function in the neonate. There are reports of increased reabsorptive rates for glucose and phosphate while for amino acids and bicarbonate the reabsorption is considerably less. Secretion of substances by the proximal straight tubule, such as para-aminohippuric acid (PAH) is also deficient. Control mechanisms for tubular functions are also immature and frequently this shows itself as an inability to cope with an excess load. For example, a baby who

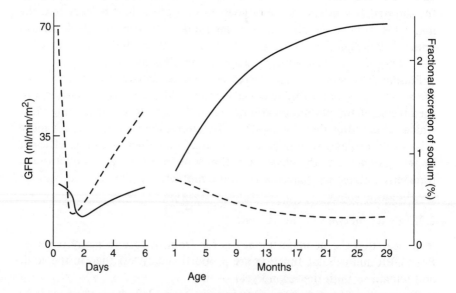

Fig. 2.12. Changes in glomerular filtration rate (GFR, ———) and fractional excretion of sodium (------) in the neonate and child. Adult values are attained after approximately 25 months.

has to excrete an excess load of salt takes much longer to do so than an adult with an equivalent load.

The inability to secrete PAH has consequences for measuring renal function. In adults 85–100 per cent of plasma PAH is extracted in a single pass through the kidneys, if the plasma concentration is sufficiently low; in infants this may be reduced to 50 per cent. Since clearance of PAH is a classical measurement equated to renal plasma flow and since it depends on complete extraction, clearance of PAH is an unreliable measure of renal plasma flow in babies.

Babies cannot concentrate their urine to the same extent as adults. Originally this was also ascribed to immaturity of the nephron, but another more reasonable explanation has now been offered. Most of the protein in the babies diet is converted to amino acids which are then used to synthesize the proteins incorporated into tissue, that is, growth. Very little is metabolized to produce urea in the liver and as a consequence plasma urea concentration in the neonate is low. Urea is essential for efficient functioning of the counter-current concentrating mechanism where it is recycled through the renal medulla. If infants are given a high protein diet or even urea in their feeds they can almost achieve the same concentrating ability as adults.

2.7.4 Micturition

The process of micturition is developed *in utero* but control is not achieved until 2–3 years of age. Reflex voiding of urine occurs whenever the stretched bladder causes stimulation of receptors in the trigone. Progressively more and more cortical control develops so that micturition occurs at a socially acceptable time.

2.7.5 Problems with renal function and fluid balance

Because the kidneys of newborn infants do not concentrate urine well there is always the threat of dehydration. This is especially so with diarrhoea and vomiting where replenishment of fluids by mouth is not possible. Any baby not taking its feed is liable to become dehydrated so that fluid balance problems frequently complicate other conditions. It is often necessary to use the intravenous route to correct dehydration.

A further problem which has been recognized in recent years is the incorrect formulation of artificial feeds for babies. Although there is no danger if feeds are made up according to the instructions a surprising number of mothers do this incorrectly. Using concentrated feeds, as well as increasing protein, fat, and carbohydrate intake, significantly increases the ingested load of ions such as sodium. Since these ions cannot be rapidly excreted their plasma concentrations may rise together with plasma osmolality, eventually causing retention of fluid and a rise in extracellular volume.

2.8 The endocrine system

Not all the endocrine organs are considered here. Many have similar functions in the fetus and adult and for many of the others information is fragmentary. Insulin and glucagon are dealt with on p. 54 and gastrointestinal hormones on p. 52. In general peptide hormones have difficulty crossing the placenta from the maternal circulation so that those which are present in the fetal circulation are usually derived from fetal endocrine glands. Some smaller peptides such as TRH may cross to a greater extent. Maternal steroids also cross to a variable extent and it must not be forgotten that oestrogen and progesterone during pregnancy require an integrated fetoplacental unit for their production. Thus, while oestriol is eventually produced in the placenta, its main precursor, dehydroepiandrosterone (DHEA), is produced by the fetal adrenal gland (see p. 65). Oestrogens and progesterone are present at such high concentrations in maternal plasma that even low permeabilities across the placenta would result in significant amounts crossing to the fetus.

2.8.1 Growth

Growth of the fetus *in utero* can be assessed by ultrasonic techniques and these give a more complete overall picture than measurements derived from infants born at various gestational ages. Weight, of course, cannot be measured by this method.

The fetus does not control its own rate of growth. Although fetal plasma growth hormone concentrations are normally higher than in neonates and adults, even anencephalic fetuses, which have no pituitary gland, grow at normal rates. Insulin-like growth factors are produced by the liver but growth hormone is not involved in their control before birth. After birth, growth hormone has its normal effects, stimulating IGF production. The very high concentration of human placental lactogen which is found in maternal plasma and is responsible for many of the maternal growth characteristics is not mirrored in fetal plasma, though there are a number of receptors for it in the fetus. How much control it exerts is not known. Prolactin does not seem to play a role. Growth of the fetus seems to be determined by genetic factors, which limit the maximum amount of growth that can occur, by placental function which controls the supply of nutrients from the mother, and by other hormones such as insulin and thyroxine. Growth is stunted if there is placental insufficiency.

After birth, the control of growth passes to the neonate although genetic and nutritional influences are still very important. Weight gain accelerates over the first weeks of postnatal life, reaches a maximum after 1–2 months and then begins to slow (Fig. 2.13). The next spurt that occurs is at puberty (see Chapter 3). Preterm babies and those which are small for the length of gestation (so-called small for dates) tend to exaggerate this postnatal growth spurt and maintain it for longer until they have effectively caught up with their genetically determined growth. Growth hormone now has its normal adult action.

2.8.2 The adrenal cortex

The fetal adrenal cortex has a distinct region known as the fetal zone which, by splitting off the C21 side chain from the steroid nucleus, produces DHEA from pregnanolone, which is itself produced in the placenta. This cleavage is important in the placental production of oestrogen. While this is important for the mother its significance in the fetus is not known. Excess production

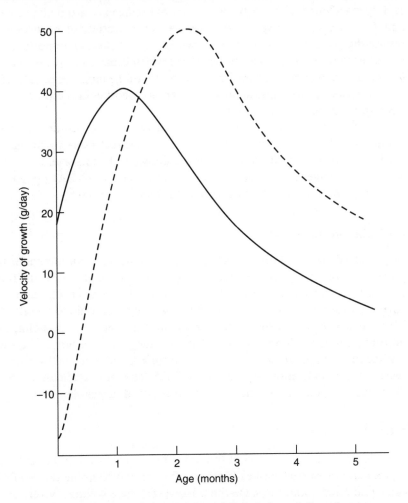

Fig. 2.13. Velocity of growth after birth in infants delivered at term (——) or before term (------).

without conversion to oestrogen can have virilizing effects. The adult zones of the adrenal cortex increase in size from mid-term onwards and produce glucocorticoids and aldosterone. Adrenocorticotrophic hormone (ACTH) stimulates both fetal and adult zones of the cortex but fetal production of ACTH may be depressed by maternal steroids crossing the placenta. Two other peptides, melanocyte-stimulating hormone (MSH) and corticotrophin-like intermediate lobe peptide (CLIP) may also play some role in stimulating secretion by the fetal zone.

The adult zone is capable of producing enough glucocorticoids and aldosterone at birth to maintain life. Since the placenta regulates salt and water balance it is unlikely that aldosterone has a significant function in the fetus, but its action in the neonate is the same as in the adult. Cortisol is rapidly inactivated in the early fetus; cortisol itself can retard both placental and fetal growth. However, the plasma concentration of cortisol rises during the last 2 months of gestation when cortisol plays an important role in maturation of many organ systems; one which is particularly noteworthy is production of surfactant by the pneumocytes of the lung (see p. 39). After birth cortisol has its usual actions through glucocorticoid receptors which develop from mid-gestation onwards.

It seems that somehow the fetal adrenal cortex is concerned with the initiation of labour but in women this seems not to be due to changes in cortisol or ACTH. Both these factors are known to be important in sheep. Metabolic changes in the placenta also seem to have a role. At present the initiating signal for human parturition still remains a mystery.

2.8.3 The adrenal medulla

The fetal adrenal medulla initially produces exclusively noradrenalin, but the proportion of adrenalin increases as gestation proceeds. What the function of these catecholamines is during fetal life is not clear although they have been suggested to constrict umbilical and placental blood vessels.

Parturition evokes a dramatic increase in noradrenalin, adrenalin, and dopamine in cord blood. The result is that they increase blood pressure, cardiac function, increase thermogenesis from BAT, and increase surfactant release and mobilization of pulmonary fluid. The more difficult the birth the higher the resulting neonatal concentrations of catecholamines.

2.8.4 The thyroid

Thyroid hormones are found in the fetus from mid-gestation onwards and thyroid-stimulating hormone (TSH) and thyrotropin-releasing factor (TRF) can be detected about the same time. However, there is little conversion of thyroxine (T_4) to tri-iodothyronine (T_3) until the third trimester but thereafter it rises to term. The production and control of thyroid hormones matures over the third trimester and early neonatal period. The precise function in fetal life is not determined but normal growth, differentiation, and development of bone, cartilage, and nervous tissue seem to require thyroid function. However, most infants with congenital hypothyroidism show no apparent signs at birth and these only develop over the succeeding weeks.

At birth TSH rises sharply and there is a dramatic increase in the conversion of T_4 to T_3. The former is probably a response to the baby's entry into a cold environment and the baby becomes selectively thyrotoxic. This probably results in an upregulation of catecholamine receptors especially in BAT and mobilization of fatty acids from fat stores. Adult levels of thyroid hormones are achieved after a few weeks.

2.9 The nervous system

Birth is of little significance in the development of the nervous system. It is possible to plot growth velocity and to give details of myelination, but all that such schedules show is that there is continuous development from conception to full maturity—birth is merely an incidental milestone along this pathway. Because of this it will be apparent that not all nervous mechanisms are present at birth—indeed reference has already been made to the incomplete development of the autonomic nervous system. Some primitive reflexes such as an upgoing planter reflex (Babinski's) sign are still present—probably because of incomplete myelination of the long tracts. Other reflexes such as tonic neck reflexes are apparent which later are suppressed by increasing corticalization; control of bowel and bladder function also develops much later.

The only ways that birth alters development of the nervous system appear to be

(1) that alterations in the cardiovascular system allow more blood to flow to the lower limbs and this enhances their growth and development; and

(2) that sensory systems of the brain are subject to an increasing number of stimuli.

This is particularly obvious in terms of vision and hearing and some time is required before the brain can interpret this plethora of new information.

Much more detailed information can be found in the *Scientific foundations of paediatrics* or *The normal child*.

Further reading

Davis, J.A. and Dobbing, J. (ed.) (1981). *Scientific foundations of paediatrics*, 2nd edn. Heinemann, London.

Fisher, D.A. (1992). Endocrinology of fetal development. In *Williams textbook of endocrinology* (ed. Wilson, J.D., Foster, D.W.), 8th edn. Saunders, Philadelphia.

Illingworth, R.S. (1991). *The normal child*, 10th edn. Churchill Livingstone, Edinburgh.

Rudolf, A.M. (1987). *Pediatrics*, 18th edn. Appleton Lange, Newark.

Spitzer, A. and Chevalier, R.L. (1992). The developing kidney and the process of growth. In *The kidney* (ed. Seldin, D.W., Giebisch, G.), 2nd edn. Raven, New York.

3

Puberty

3.1 Puberty—its definition and timing

Puberty is often defined as that time over which the ability to reproduce is achieved. The word *puberty* is derived from the Latin *pubescere*, which means to be covered with hair. Neither this derivation nor a definition based on reproductive capacity can describe adequately the complex physiological processes involved. During puberty, the body grows to reach adult stature and physical maturation, the reproductive organs mature to become fully functional in producing mature ova and spermatozoa, and psychological changes occur related to both reproductive ability and body growth. Development of the secondary sexual characteristics, rapid skeletal growth to final adult stature, and changes in both lean body mass and fat distribution all occur. These must be precisely controlled and co-ordinated.

The timing of puberty varies considerably (Fig. 3.1). The first signs normally occur between 8 and 13 years of age in girls, and between 9 and 14 years in boys. Girls complete puberty in a mean of 4.2 years (range 1.5–6.0 years), while in boys it takes a mean of 3.5 years (range 2.0–4.5 years).

3.1.1 Physical characterization

In girls, development of secondary sexual characteristics involves enlargement of the ovaries, uterus, vagina, labia and breasts, the growth of pubic hair, and the change to a typical female body shape. The vagina increases in length and continues to enlarge until menarche (the first menstruation). The mons pubis increases in size by fat deposition and the labia become larger. The uterus grows during early puberty by enlargement of the myometrium, though the endometrium does not commence development until the onset of the secondary sexual characteristics. The breasts develop in defined stages

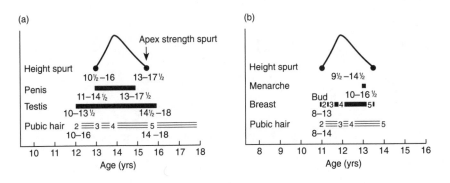

Fig. 3.1. Sequence of secondary sexual development in British (a) males and (b) females. The range of ages and stages of puberty are indicated. From Marshall, W.A. and Tanner, J.M. (1970). *Arch. Dis. Child*, **45**, 13.

in a mean of 4 years, while pubic hair takes approximately 2.5 years to grow to completion. Axillary hair also grows and the associated apocrine glands begin to function, sometimes leading to acne (a major cause of concern in adolescents). Menarche occurs at the peak of the body growth spurt and within 2 years or so of the initiation of breast growth. Thereafter, the menstrual cycles in adolescent girls show considerable variation in length; approximately 90 per cent of these cycles are anovulatory. In girls, pubic hair and breast development are used to define the different stages of puberty in a series of stages (Marshall and Tanner, 1969).

In boys, secondary sexual development involves both pubic hair growth and genital development. Testicular enlargement occurs first, resulting in an increase in volume from 4–6 to 15–25 ml; it is followed by phallic enlargement (from 6.2 cm stretched flaccid length to 13.2 cm in the adult). In conjunction with penile growth, the seminal vesicles, prostate, and bulbourethral glands enlarge and develop, in order to provide suitable secretions for sperm transport. After genital development begins, pubic hair generally starts to appear and takes a mean of 2.6 years to complete its growth. However, the development of facial and axillary hair is very variable, beginning at approximately 15 years of age. The larynx also enlarges and this brings about the deepening of the voice characteristic of puberty. In boys,

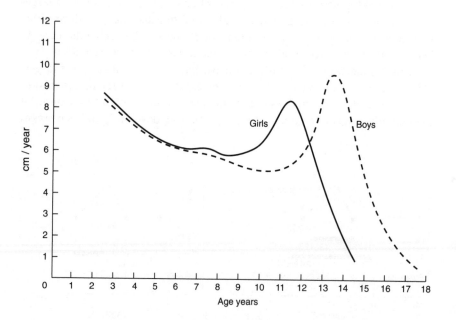

Fig. 3.2. The height velocity for chronological age (CA) for healthy North American (a) boys and (b) girls. From Tanner, J.M. and Davies, P.W. (1985). *J. Pediatr.*, **107**, 317.

pubic hair development and genital development is also divided into different stages (1–5) to identify the progress of puberty (Marshall and Tanner, 1970).

3.1.2 Body growth in puberty

Paradoxically, puberty both promotes body growth and limits ultimate body height. There is a significant increase in height velocity (the rate of body height increase per year) and the rate of skeletal maturation is speeded up, resulting in epiphysial cartilage fusion. The growth spurt or increase in height velocity, occurs earlier in girls than boys (Fig. 3.2), though the later onset in boys results in a longer growth period. In boys and girls, both leg and trunk growth contribute to the overall increase in height. Leg growth precedes trunk growth by approximately 1 year. The sequence of leg growth is feet first, then calves and thighs. Similarly, growth of hands and forearms precedes that of the upper arms. The growth spurt reaches a maximum at stage 4 in boys (7–12 cm/year), but at stage 3 in girls (6–11 cm/year). In view of the bone growth occurring, skeletal age may be used to reflect the degree of physiological maturation during puberty. This is often termed bone age, which is defined by a series of radiographical standard images of bone development. These images are used in relation to the bone growth of an individual child as well as to predict how much of the child's growth remains to occur and what the final height will be.

3.1.3 Changes in body shape and composition

Before puberty, boys and girls have a very similar body shape and composition; these are altered considerably during puberty. Lean body mass increases during the early stages of puberty, mainly reflecting an increase in muscle mass. This muscle mass increases in girls up to menarche and then decreases. In boys, muscle mass continues to increase throughout puberty, to reach values much higher than those in girls. Bone width and muscle width increase in boys, usually accompanied by a loss of body fat. In girls, fat mass increases, especially in late puberty, to values eventually almost twice those found in boys. As part of the increase in lean body mass, there is co-ordinated growth of the organs such as heart, liver, lungs, and kidneys.

3.2 Hormonal changes during puberty

Co-ordination of the complex events of puberty requires a very precise and well-timed means of regulation. This is achieved via specific hormonal systems, whose blood-borne chemical messengers act alone and in conjunction with other hormones, to control body growth and development. A major and essential part of the hormonal control comes from the gonadal steroids, which are regulated by the pituitary gonadotrophins and hypo-thalamic gonadotrophin-releasing hormone (GnRH). GnRH is released from the median eminence of the hypothalamus and is carried in the hypophysial portal blood to the anterior pituitary, where it stimulates the release of the two gonadotrophins, luteinizing hormone (LH) and follicle-stimulating hormone (FSH). These, in turn, influence secretion of the gonadal steroids (oestrogens, progestagens, and androgens). This con-trolled hormonal sequence is initiated by pulsatile release of GnRH: pulse frequency and amplitude are varied during the stages of pubertal develop-ment by a pulse generator whose rhythmical activity originates in the hypo-thalamic arcuate nucleus.

3.2.1 Changes in secretion of the hypothalamic–pituitary–gonadal hormones

In boys, the most important gonadal steroid is testosterone, although dihydrotestosterone and oestradiol-17β are also important. Testosterone is the primary stimulant for development of the reproductive organs, as well as for body growth. Testosterone secretion increases dramatically during stages 2–5 of puberty (see Fig. 3.3). Initially, the increased secretion occurs at night, but with advancing puberty, the enhanced secretion occurs throughout day and night. Testosterone binds to the sex hormone-binding globulin (SHBG) in plasma. As a result, only approximately 30 per cent of circulating testosterone is free and physiologically active. Plasma SHBG concentrations decrease during puberty, since androgens reduce SHBG synthesis and this will permit more free testosterone to be available for its growth-promoting actions. To enhance androgen secretion, both FSH and LH release are increased during puberty (see Fig. 3.3): in accord with the pattern of androgen secretion, there is first a nocturnal increase in gonado-trophin release, which ultimately also occurs during the day. An increased GnRH pulse amplitude every 60–90 min is responsible for the initial nocturnal gonadotrophin release and the gonadotrophin peaks become more regular during daytime as puberty progresses, until the diurnal rhythm disappears in adulthood.

In girls, the hormonal mechanisms are very similar to those in boys: between 6 and 9 years of age, gonadotrophin secretion begins to increase gradually, as a result of increased GnRH secretion (see Fig. 3.3). Pulsatile GnRH release starts during sleep (between approximately 01.00 and 06.00), thereby enhancing gonadotrophin secretion and, ultimately, oestradiol secretion (Fig. 3.3). Pituitary sensitivity to GnRH and ovarian sensitivity to gonadotrophins both increase as the secretion of GnRH, LH, and FSH change from nocturnal into nocturnal and daytime patterns. Gonado-trophin secretion is enhanced during early puberty in a monthly cyclical pattern which, in turn, stimulates cyclical oestrogen secretion and, hence, growth of the reproductive organs. Eventually, during late puberty, the monthly (menstrual) cycle pattern of secretion is established, with mid-cycle LH and FSH peaks. This requires the positive feedback effect of oestrogens to have developed so as to generate the increased GnRH release necessary for the mid-cycle gonadotrophin peaks. Progesterone acts synergistically with oestrogens to increase GnRH pulse amplitude and the pituitary responsiveness to GnRH. SHBG increases during puberty in girls as a result of oestrogen stimulating its production. Since androgens bind well to SHBG, their effects in girls are minimized.

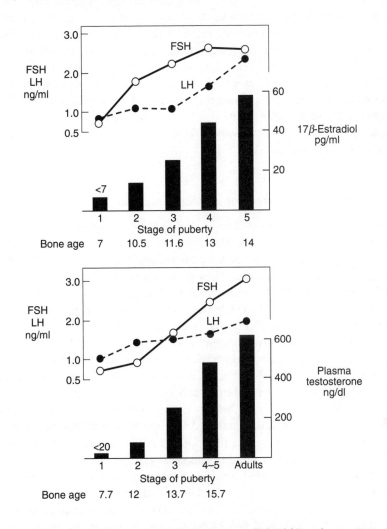

Fig. 3.3. Mean plasma LH, FSH, and oestradiol (girls) and testosterone (boys) correlated with age and stage of puberty. From Grumbach, M.M. (1975). In *Puberty* (ed. Berenberg, S.R.), Martinus Nijhoff, Dordrecht, The Netherlands.

3.2.2 Changes in adrenal steroid secretion

Between 6 and 8 years of age, the adrenal cortex starts to secrete increased amounts of androgens, especially dehydroepiandrosterone, DHA (see Fig. 3.4). This change in adrenal steroid secretion is usually termed *adrenarche* and is eventually accompanied by the appearance of pubic hair and axillary hair. The increased adrenal androgen output is independent of either adrenocorticotrophin (ACTH) or cortisol secretion. Although the timing of the DHA increase is variable, it occurs before the observed increase in gonadotrophin and, hence, gonadal steroid secretion. It results in a transient increase in both bone maturation and linear growth. Perhaps, an as yet unidentified pituitary factor is responsible for stimulating DHA secretion, since it is ACTH-independent. The increased adrenal androgens may also regulate GnRH release, as well as decreasing SHBG levels in boys. These two actions together would facilitate the pubertal process, ultimately allowing more free testosterone to be available for the stimulation of body growth. However, adrenarche is not essential for puberty to occur, since some children with precocious puberty (see later) have not reached or undergone adrenarche.

3.2.3 Changes in the secretion of other hormones

Among the many physical changes during puberty, the growth spurt can be easily recognized (Fig. 3.2). However, the precise endocrine environment producing this spurt has not been identified. After the onset of puberty, linear body growth increases, then decreases rapidly to zero as a result of epiphyseal fusion. Obviously, growth hormone (GH) and insulin-like growth factor-1 (IGF-1), which mediates the growth-promoting actions of GH, must be involved. Plasma levels of IGF-1 rise during puberty in association with the growth spurt and decline to adult levels thereafter: these increased plasma concentrations occur earlier in girls than in boys. Correlation of the IGF-1 concentrations with GH release is much more difficult in view of the pulsatile and circadian patterns of GH release. Growth hormone-releasing hormone concentrations in plasma increase from mid-puberty and the increased GH plasma concentration (mean 24 h value), GH pulse area, and number of GH pulses per 24 h all correlate with the growth spurt in late puberty (stages 3–4).

These increases in IGF-1 and GH have been compared with other hormones' secretion during puberty. The gonadotrophins show a progressive increase in secretion throughout. By contrast, GH concentrations are highest at stage 2–3 in girls and 4–5 in boys, while prolactin concentrations are highest at stage 2–3 in boys and 4–5 in girls. Pulse periodicities for GH and prolactin are 150–180 min in girls and 180 min in boys; gonadotrophin pulse period rises from 180 to 90 min as puberty progresses in both boys and girls. Pulses of LH and prolactin follow GH pulses with a lag of 30–75 min for LH and 30 min for prolactin. LH, FSH, and prolactin pulses are all in phase with each other. This would suggest that, at least for the anterior pituitary hormones, some degree of co-ordination of release exists. Since each pulse of secretion is under hypothalamic regulation, control of the pulse generator in the hypothalamus may be the site of this co-ordination.

3.3 Psychological changes during puberty

Although brain growth is largely complete before puberty, major behavioural changes occur, indicative of altered central nervous system function in relation to puberty. The most obvious are those related to reproduction: attraction to members of the opposite sex, display patterns to enhance attraction, and the development of libido (or sexual desire). Neurones throughout the brain possess receptors for sex steroids. Because of their lipid solubility and ease of passage through the blood–brain barrier, sex steroids can therefore directly influence neuronal activity. In view of the presence of GnRH and its receptors extrahypothalamically within the brain and its ability to control mating behaviour in animals, this polypeptide may co-ordinate both the hormonal and behavioural changes in puberty.

Other behavioural changes occur during puberty. Bouts of aggression and depression are often experienced, which may be a reflection of changes in brain function caused by the changes in either hormonal secretion (gonadal steroids) or in neurotransmitter systems. For example, dopamine content, tyrosine hydroxylase activity, and β-endorphin content in the hypothalamus are all changed during puberty in rats. These exemplify the potential for altered central nervous system function, as do the changes in appetite and feeding behaviour. Appetite is markedly increased to provide the energy and materials necessary for growth, in direct correlation with the physiological and metabolic demands made on the body to bring about sustained body development and growth. All these behavioural changes require considerable tolerance and understanding on the part of parents whose children are experiencing the various stages of puberty.

3.4 Physiological and metabolic demands of puberty

During the years of puberty, the lungs, heart and circulatory system, gastrointestinal tract, and kidneys must all develop to facilitate the progressive increase in body growth, until they in turn reach adult status. Such processes of growth and development are gradual, being related directly to the nutritional and metabolic requirements of puberty. It is likely that gonadal steroids, GH and IGF-1, insulin, thyroid hormones, adrenal steroids, and other potential growth factors are involved in organ growth. Organs grow under the influence of GH and IGF-1. For example, the heart grows significantly in size during acromegaly; therefore, both GH and IGF-1 may be involved in overall body growth. The haematocrit also increases during puberty, indicating enhanced erythropoietin secretion to increase red blood cell formation.

The metabolic demands of puberty must also be considered. Body growth and development require not only energy, but also sufficient amino acids, carbohydrates, and free fatty acids to achieve the sustained body growth. As a consequence, an enhanced, balanced diet is essential and appetite is increased throughout puberty. Often, the metabolic demands can outweigh input and transient hypoglycaemia results. The metabolic demands of puberty can also provide a trigger for the occurrence of juvenile-onset (Type 1) diabetes mellitus in those children with a predisposition for this condition.

3.5 Control of puberty

The control of puberty must involve mechanisms which regulate gonado-trophin and gonadal steroid secretion. The observed increase in LH, FSH, and gonadal steroid release infers a preceding increase in hypothalamic secretion of GnRH. How the hypothalamic response is triggered remains to be determined, but it appears to require multiple inputs to the hypothalamus such as nutritional state, metabolic rate, stress, and hormonal feedback mechanisms. However, neuroendocrine control of gonadal steroids is not the only important mechanism: the increased release of GH, prolactin, TSH, and ACTH which is necessary during puberty must be mediated hypothalamically. There must be some stimulus or series of stimuli, to trigger the hypothalamus into a co-ordinated, increased release of its regu-latory hormones, which in turn increases secretion of the relevant pituitary and other hormones involved in controlling the physical events of puberty. Various suggestions have been made about the nature of this stimulus, including the attainment of a critical height:body weight ratio, a gradual change in the threshold of steroid feedback with age during puberty, and the role of adequate sleep to produce pulsatile gonadotrophin secretion. None of these is sufficient to explain the complex control of various hormonal systems which must actually occur during puberty.

3.5.1 Hypothalamic regulation of gonadotrophin secretion

During early puberty, pulsatile gonadotrophin release has been observed, initially during sleep and, subsequently, during the daytime as well. This results from increased pulsatile GnRH secretion from the median eminence of the hypothalamus, which is regulated by a pulse generator located in the mediobasal hypothalamic region (probably the arcuate nucleus). GnRH pulse frequency and amplitude must be increased progressively during puberty to achieve the gradual elevation of gonadotrophin and gonadal steroid secretion; the increased secretory activity is produced by maturation of the hypothalamus and its neuronal connections.

Central to the control of GnRH release is a series of interactions in the mediobasal hypothalamus (MBH) between dopamine, β-endorphin, and GnRH (see Fig. 3.4). Dopamine stimulates GnRH release, whereas β-endorphin inhibits its release. At the same time, dopamine can activate β-endorphin-containing nerve cells, which, in turn, inhibit dopamine release. Dopaminergic neuronal activity increases during puberty in rats: there is an increase in tyrosine hydroxylase activity in the median eminence and migration of dopaminergic neurones from the median eminence to the

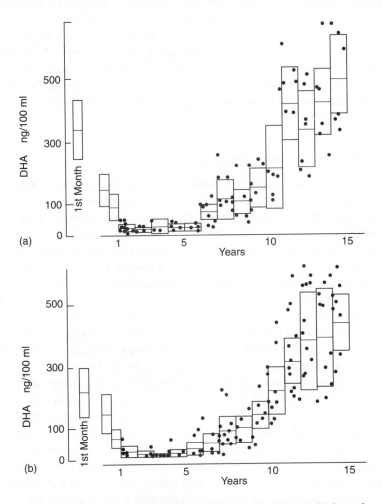

Fig. 3.4. Plasma concentrations of DHA in (a) girls and (b) boys from ages 1 to 15 years. From de Peretti, G. and Forrest, M. (1976). *J. Clin. Endocrinol. Metab.*, **43**, 982.

arcuate nucleus, which seems to activate both the GnRH- and β-endorphin-containing neurones. Gonadal steroids, notably oestradiol, can decrease GnRH release by effects on both dopamine- and β-endorphin-containing neurones and this is possibly the way in which progressive changes in hypothalamic sensitivity to gonadal steroids occur. One may postulate gradual steroid activation of dopaminergic neurones, then stimulation of relatively quiescent GnRH and β-endorphin neurones, until the β-endorphin gradually inhibits both dopamine and GnRH release. Maturation of the pulse generator may require stimulation by neurotrophic factors such as nerve growth factor, transforming growth factor α, or IGF-1. For example, there is now evidence of IGF-1 having the ability to activate pulsatile GnRH release in puberty. Nutritional factors are also involved, since starvation inhibits pulsatile LH secretion, perhaps via a stress-related response involving β-endorphin. To date, numerous potential mechanisms might be involved in pubertal maturation of the hypothalamus. All, or some of, these may interact via the MBH dopamine–GnRH–β-endorphin system. It is much more likely that a combination of these factors will gradually influence GnRH secretion and co-ordinate the release of other hormones which have a role in puberty.

3.5.2 Body composition, stress, and puberty

Some clues to the mechanisms controlling puberty may be obtained from abnormalities, such as precocious and delayed puberty and other clinical conditions capable of altering puberty (dwarfism, diabetes mellitus, and anorexia nervosa). One hypothesis concerns the attainment of a critical body weight or, more correctly, a body height to weight ratio before reproductive capacity can be reached. This will require a progressive increase in overall body growth, with accompanying increases in food intake and in fat and muscle deposition. These may be better expressed in terms of the changes observed in lean body mass and adipose tissue (especially in girls at menarche), which must reach critical values before reproduction can occur. In starvation and anorexia nervosa, body weight decreases and menstrual cycles stop, resulting in secondary amenorrhoea. Once body weight increases again, the menstrual cycles restart, tending to confirm the necessity for a particular body weight or composition for reproduction to occur in women at least. Similarly, in juvenile-onset (Type 1) diabetes, the lack of body growth and development caused by the insulin deficit may delay puberty. These are all stressful clinical conditions, which could be mediated via the release of corticotrophin-releasing factor (CRF). CRF is known to inhibit food intake, to release β-endorphin, and to inhibit both gonadotrophin secretion and reproductive behaviour by direct neuronal actions. Thus it can contribute to the inhibitory mechanisms acting to slow pubertal development.

3.6 Abnormalities of puberty

Although puberty occurs normally in most children, it may happen much earlier than anticipated (*precocious puberty*) or be later than expected (*delayed puberty*). The causes of both conditions are many and varied, but the occurrence of delayed and precocious puberty can be recognized by reference to the normal values of body growth and development of secondary sexual characteristics. The design of therapy for the abnormalities now relies on what limited knowledge there is about the normal control of puberty.

3.6.1 Precocious puberty—its causes and management

Development of secondary sexual characteristics before 8 years of age in girls or 9 years in boys, constitutes precocious puberty. Many causes have been identified: these are classified as central and peripheral precocious puberty, variations of normal pubertal development, and contrasexual development. Central precocious puberty can result from damage to the brain through tumours, abesses, meningitis, and head trauma, whereas peripheral precocious puberty can be due to ovarian, testicular, or adrenal tumours. In central precocious puberty, premature pulsatile GnRH release brings about pulsatile gonadotrophin secretion and an increase in gonadal steroid release. Peripheral precocious puberty occurs via either extra-pituitary gonadotrophin or gonadal steroid secretion in the absence of hypothalamic or pituitary control. Management of both types of precocious puberty relies on treatment of the underlying cause, such as surgery or radiation therapy of a tumour. In the absence of a known cause, the therapy must be designed to suppress gonadal steroid secretion selectively and effectively, to stop premature sexual maturation, and to ensure attainment of normal skeletal height despite a more rapid, abnormal growth rate. For central precocious puberty, medroxyprogesterone acetate can be used to suppress gonadotrophin secretion, although this steroid does have some adverse reactions. Current therapy involves the use of GnRH agonists, long-acting analogues of the parent decapeptide molecule, which have been modified at positions six and ten to enhance stability to enzymic degradation and to improve receptor binding. If given in continuous large doses (subcutaneously or by depot preparation) the agonists have a paradoxical effect of down-regulating pituitary GnRH receptors, and so reduce gonadotrophin and gonadal steroid secretion. Close continuous monitoring of such a patient is necessary to assess the treatment's effectiveness. For peripheral precocious puberty, androgen antagonists, testolactone (a competitive inhibitor of the enzyme converting androgen to oestrogen), and keto-conazole (an inhibitor of testosterone synthesis) are used.

3.6.2 Delayed puberty—its causes and management

Delayed puberty is defined in any girl of 13 years of age or boy of 14 years, showing no signs of pubertal development and with a shorter than predicted stature. Many causes are possible but, in general, decreased secretion of either GnRH or gonadotrophins may be responsible. Decreased secretion can, in turn, be caused by tumours such as craniopharyngioma, by isolated hormone deficiency (gonadotrophins or GH), by hypothyroidism, or by radiation therapy, which can damage pituitary function. If the cause is diagnosed as gonadotrophin deficiency, long-term pulsatile GnRH therapy (pulses every 90–120 min for several years) can be used to replace lost pituitary stimulation. Human chorionic gonadotrophin or long-acting sex steroids may also be utilized. For patients with a co-existing GH deficiency, genetically engineered human GH may also be given. Continuous observations of the development of secondary sexual characteristics and of body growth rate, are necessary to ensure that an appropriate dosage is being used effectively.

3.6.3 Other causes of pubertal abnormalities

In view of the complex hormonal interactions involved in the normal regulation of puberty, it is not unexpected that pubertal abnormalities can be associated with other endocrine disorders. These include GH deficiency (hypopituitary dwarfism), juvenile-onset (Type 1) diabetes mellitus, hypothyroidism, and anorexia nervosa. In each case, the primary deficiency is not directly related to the hypothalamus–pituitary–gonadal axis, but it can influence the normal course of growth and development associated with puberty, through a hormonal deficiency or imbalance.

3.7 Puberty as a life stage

Puberty represents a vital stage during which physical adulthood (in terms of body size, composition, and reproductive ability) is achieved by a series of active, well controlled steps of growth and development. Without these physiological and psychological changes, reproduction would not be possible. Puberty is a gradual process, drawn out over 6 years or more, to permit growth without undue stress or strain on any body system and to allow successful reproduction to occur. As such, the mechanisms for controlling puberty must be well co-ordinated via the central nervous system and the hypothalamus in particular. Despite an increasing knowledge of the changes in hormonal secretion during puberty, much remains to be learned about the precise mechanisms regulating hormonal release in the numerous interacting systems and how these relate to the changes occurring in body growth and development. Although the physical events are well defined, how they are brought about is poorly understood. However, the current state of knowledge has permitted a better understanding of abnormalities related to puberty, as well as the development of therapies to be applied successfully to these abnormalities. Such abnormalities provide an equally valuable insight into how the normal mechanisms controlling puberty can be disturbed. It is hoped that future research will provide a much clearer understanding of the complexities that define and regulate puberty.

Further reading

Giusti, M. and Cavagnaro, P. (1991). Update on pulsatile luteinizing hormone-releasing hormone therapy in males with idiopathic hypogonadotropichypo-gonadism and delayed puberty. *Journal of Endocrinological Investigation*, **14**, 419–29.

Marshall, W.A. and Tanner, J.M. (1969). Variations in the pattern of pubertal changes in girls. *Archives of Diseases of Childhood*, **44**, 291–303.

Marshall, W.A. and Tanner, J.M. (1970). Variations in the pattern of pubertal changes in boys. *Archives of Diseases of Childhood*, **45**, 13–32.

Ojeda, S.R. (1991). The mystery of mammalian puberty: how much do we know? *Perspectives in Biology and Medicine*, **34**, 365–83.

Petersen, A.C. (1988). Adolescent development. *Annual Review of Psychology*, **39**, 583–607.

Rasmussen, D. (1991). The interaction between mediobasal dopaminergic and endorphinergic neuronal systems as a key regulator of reproduction: an hypothesis. *Journal of Endocrinological Investigation*, **14**, 323–52.

Styne, D.M. (1990). Puberty. In *Basic and clinical endocrinology*, (ed. F. Greenspan, Lange), pp. 519–42.

Styne, D.M. (ed.) (1991). Puberty and its disorders. *Endocrinology and Metabolism*, **20** (1), 1–235.

Wheeler, M.D. and Styne, D.M. (1991). Drug treatment in precocious puberty. *Drugs*, **41**, 717–28.

4

The menopause

4.1 The menopause—its definition and timing

The menopause is that stage in a woman's life during which menstruation ceases and there are no further menstrual cycles, effectively ending reproductive function. It is also referred to as 'the change of life' or *climacteric*, which describes the considerable alterations in a woman's physiology caused by dynamic modifications to reproductive hormone secretion and the cessation of menstruation. Because these changes are usually spread over a number of years, it is possible to subdivide the menopause into a *perimenopausal time* prior to and immediately after the loss of menstruation and a *post-menopausal time* constituting the rest of a woman's life. Surgical removal of the ovaries (ovariectomy) will also result in the menopause.

The menopause occurs within the age range 41–59 years, with a mean of 50.8 years in the UK, though it is often difficult to establish the precise timing of the last menstrual cycle. It is not unknown for irregular menstrual cycles to occur for 2–3 years, complicating determination of the exact timing. Whether there is a male equivalent remains to be confirmed: men have the ability to retain reproductive capacity until well into their eighties, though they are less sexually active and their androgen levels decline with increasing age from 40–50 years onwards.

4.2 Physical characteristics of the menopause

The most obvious event of the menopause is the complete loss of menstrual cycles and accompanying menstruation. However, there are many other physiological effects. In 10 per cent of women, these may be sufficiently subtle to be unapparent, but in most, they are noticeable and for 10–15 per cent of women, they are so severe that they will interfere with normal, daily activities.

The most commonly reported change in the perimenopausal years is the occurrence of hot flushes, sudden but intense feelings of heat in the chest, neck, and face, accompanied by sweating and some discomfort. The flushes last 3–5 min, they are more common at night, and they may include other diverse symptoms such as heart palpitations, nausea, headache, irritability, anxiety, and sleeplessness. These vasomotor changes may be due to episodic release of adrenalin, since they are very similar to those experienced by patients with phaeochromocytomas (tumours of the adrenal medulla). At the time of a hot flush, heart rate, skin blood flow, and skin temperature all increase (Fig. 4.1), indicating a transient peripheral vasodilatation. This can be accompanied by release of a variety of hormones including LH, GnRH, adrenalin, cortisol, ACTH, β-endorphin, GH, and neurotensin. The most interesting of these hormonal changes is the correlation between the hot flushes and increased pulsatile LH release (Fig. 4.2), which itself results from changes in GnRH release. Hot flushes appear to be a physiological response to a sudden, but transient, downward resetting of the hypo-thalamic thermoregulatory set-point. The mechanism involved is not known. One current hypothesis is that declining plasma oestrogen concentrations reduce hypothalamic catecholamine concentrations, leading to a vasomotor instability and GnRH release.

During the menopause, the cyclical changes in breast volume apparent during the menstrual cycle no longer occur. The breasts become smaller, their fibrous tissue increases, and glandular tissue decreases. The nipples are smaller, flatter, and no longer erectile. Since 80 per cent of breast cancers

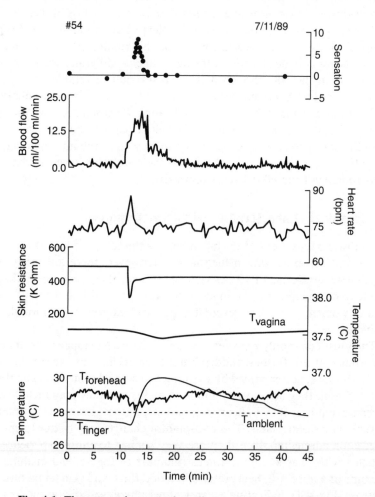

Fig. 4.1. Thermoregulatory and cardiovascular changes during a typical hot flush at an ambient temperature of 28°C. Subjective sensation, blood flow (finger), heart rate, skin resistance (chest), internal body temperature (vagina), and skin temperatures (forehead, finger) are depicted. From Kronenberg, F. In: Flint, M. *et al.* (1990) (ed.) *Ann. NY Acad. Sci.*, **592**, 1.

occur in women over 40 years of age, regular breast examination should be undertaken. With suitable training, self-examination at monthly intervals is highly recommended. These same procedures must be undertaken before and during hormone replacement therapy (HRT), which is becoming more widely prescribed both peri- and post-menopausally.

The vaginal epithelium is also influenced menopausally, because it is normally very sensitive to changes in oestrogen concentrations. There is reduced maturation, reduced vaginal fluid secretion, and an increase in vaginal pH (from pH 4.0–5.5 to 6.0–8.0). The reduced vaginal secretion (dyspareuria) and very easily traumatized vaginal epithelium may lead to painful sexual intercourse. Similar regression of the cervical epithelium occurs. The uterus and fallopian tubes become atrophic, so that uterine weight is decreased from approximately 120 to 60 g or less. All these effects are as a direct result of reduced oestrogen production by the ovaries (see later).

Because the skin is also directly influenced by oestrogens, it becomes more easily traumatized with the menopause. It is drier due to reduced activity in the sweat and sebaceous glands and wound healing is much slower. The skin shows a more wrinkled appearance, the scalp hair thins, and there may be increased facial hair and areas of pigmentation. Skin collagen also decreases, probably reflecting overall body collagen losses and this causes skin sagging. The network of papillary capillaries responsible for

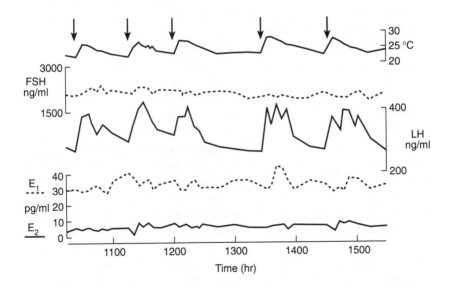

Fig. 4.2. Serial measurements of finger temperature and serum follicle-stimulating hormone (FSH), luteinizing hormone (LH), oestrone (E_1), and oestradiol (E_2) in an individual subject. From Meldrum, D.R. (1980). *J. Clin. Endocrin. Metab.*, **50**, 685.

skin microcirculation also declines after the menopause and results in reduced thickness of both the dermis and epidermis.

One of the most serious physical changes associated with the menopause is osteoporosis. An imbalance appears between formation and resorption of bone, resulting in enhanced bone resorption. The osteoblasts fail to repair this defect and there is a consequent increase in bone fragility, which is manifested as an increased incidence of bone fractures (especially hip fracture, Colles's fracture, and vertebral crush fracture). The increased calcium loss from bone produces a slight elevation of plasma calcium, but there is no clear evidence whether the hormones regulating calcium balance (calcitonin, parathyroid hormone, and 1,25-dihydroxy-vitamin D_3) are altered post-menopausally. Perhaps increased production of other factors known to cause bone resorption, such as prostaglandin E_2 and interleukin 1, may be involved during the menopause and there could be reduced production (or effectiveness) of factors enhancing bone formation, such as insulin-like growth factor-1 (IGF-1) and transforming growth factor-β (TGF-β). IGF-1 (and GH) plasma concentrations decrease with increasing age and it is possible that a series of hormonal events, rather than a single hormonal change, is responsible for the osteoporosis. Measurement of bone density enables the assessment of menopausal changes: bone density has been found to decrease with increasing age in women and the decrease is accelerated at the menopause. Bone density measurement also permits an appreciation of the effectiveness of various therapies menopausally including HRT, increased calcium intake, combined calcium/sodium fluoride treatment, and exercise regimes.

Throughout reproductive life, the ovaries are active in the menstrual cycle, producing a mature ovum in conjunction with cyclical ovarian steroid secretion patterns. The menopause marks the cessation of these cyclical events. The ovaries decrease in size by up to 70 per cent, with the outer cortical zone depleted of growing and maturing follicles. From mid-fetal life onwards, the ovaries lose follicles steadily, from approximately 10^6 fetally to 10^3/ovary at 40 years of age, a decline which is relatively linear in nature (Fig. 4.3). The rate of follicle loss from 40 years onwards is much more rapid, with no follicles found post-menopausally (50 years and over). Why the rate of loss increases at this time is unknown, though FSH secretion is selectively enhanced and this gonadotrophin could cause a greater proportion of primordial follicles to enter the growing pool of follicles and then the follicles become atretic. Reduced blood flow to and fibrosis of the ovarian cortex also occurs. Surface epithelium inclusion cysts and papillary projections become more obvious in the post-menopausal ovaries, at a time when there is very clear depletion of oocytes. Both the ovarian cortex and medulla are now made up of stromal cells and are still capable of steroid production. Testosterone and androstenedione are the major steroids produced, with only minor amounts of oestradiol, oestrone, and progesterone. Hence, the ovaries change from organs rich in follicles and secreting oestrogens and progestagens cyclically, to those containing stroma cells secreting androgens in a non-cyclical manner.

A potentially serious consequence of the menopause is a doubling in the incidence rate of coronary heart disease post-menopausally. Several factors may contribute. The haematocrit increases from 37–39 to 42–45 per cent, with a consequent increased blood viscosity and increased resistance to blood flow. There are also changes in lipid metabolism. Pre-menopausal women have increased high-density lipoprotein (HDL) concentrations and decreased low-density lipoprotein (LDL) in their plasma, when compared with either post-menopausal women or with men. These lipoproteins transport lipids such as triglycerides and cholesterol through the plasma. In general, the more HDL there is available, the more unesterified cholesterol can be transported to the liver to be redigested. When less HDL is available, cholesterol deposition in blood vessels becomes more likely and, hence, the potential for heart disease increases. Oestrogens maintain increased HDL concentrations, so a reduction in their secretion will obviously change the amount of HDL available.

4.3 Psychological changes associated with the menopause

Despite considerable investigation, there is still no clear evidence to support the occurrence of specific psychological changes associated with the meno-

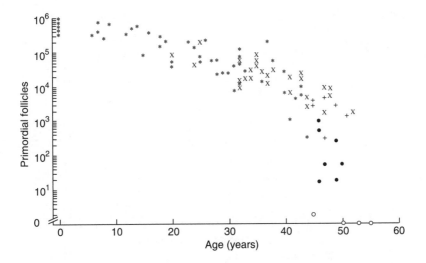

Fig. 4.3. The relationship between age and primordial follicle number is compared using data from four studies. Follicle depletion appears to accelerate in the decade preceding menopause. From Richardson, S.J. and Nelson, J.F. In: Flint, M. *et al.* (1990) (ed.) *Ann. NY Acad. Sci.*, **592**, 1.

pause. Some, but not all, women have reported symptoms including irritability, depression, anxiety, sleeplessness, headaches, tiredness, dizzy spells, joint and back pains, and palpitations. It is continually debated whether these symptoms are directly related to the hormonal and physical changes at menopause or whether they are related to cultural, social, and family factors, which can influence a woman's mental health at this stage of life. Although there is no specific psychiatric syndrome associated with the menopause, it is still possible that the physiological changes could affect the vulnerability of some women to psychiatric disorders. For example, reduced binding of ovarian hormones to steroid receptors throughout the brain is a potential source of change in central nervous system function.

4.4 Hormonal changes during the menopause

The menopause results from a gradual loss of ovarian function. Ovarian steroid secretion is altered very significantly and, as a result, other changes in hormone secretion are brought about. For example, secretion of the gonadotrophins (LH and FSH), IRH, and inhibin are all known to be influenced.

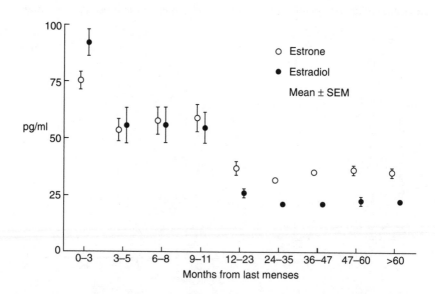

Fig. 4.4. Concentrations (pg/ml) of oestrone and oestradiol related to time from last menses in a group of 78 peri- and post-menopausal women. From Longcope, C. In: Flint, M. *et al.* (1990) (ed.) *Ann. NY Acad. Sci.*, **592**, 1.

Table 4.1. Concentrations of some steroids in 55 pre-menopausal women (under 40 y) and 54 post-menopausal women (over 60 y). From Longcope, C. In: Flint, M. *et al.* (1990) (ed.) *Ann. NY Acad. Sci.*, **592**, 1.

		<40 yr	>60 yr
Androstenedione	ng/ml	1.3 ±0.1[a,b]	0.50±0.04[c]
Testosterone	ng/ml	0.31±0.02[b]	0.19±0.02[c]
Estrone	pg/ml	57 ±4[b]	27 ±2[c]
Estradiol	pg/ml	69 ±6[b]	11 ±1[c]

[a] Mean±SEM.
[b,c] Difference between means is significant, $p < 0.01$.

4.4.1 Changes in steroid secretion

From the time of the last menstruation, plasma concentrations of oestradiol and oestrone (Fig. 4.4) and progesterone (Fig. 4.5) decline over the following year or more. Androstenedione and testosterone concentrations also decrease. Peripheral aromatization (that is, the conversion of androgens to oestrogens) in tissues such as the liver, skeletal muscle, kidney, adipose tissue, brain, and hair follicles is significantly increased post-menopausally in the case of both androstenedione to oestrone and testosterone to oestradiol (Table 4.1). Aromatization now becomes the primary source of oestrogens, rather than the ovaries themselves.

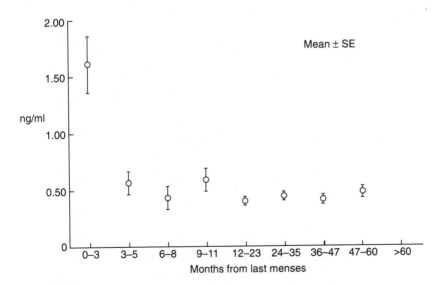

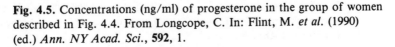

Fig. 4.5. Concentrations (ng/ml) of progesterone in the group of women described in Fig. 4.4. From Longcope, C. In: Flint, M. *et al.* (1990) (ed.) *Ann. NY Acad. Sci.*, **592**, 1.

4.4.2 **Changes in gonadotrophin and other hormones' secretion**

In the 2–3 years after the menopause, plasma concentrations of LH and, especially, FSH increase (Fig. 4.6). These changes result directly from the removal of the oestrogen/progestagen negative feedback of both the hypothalamus and anterior pituitary and a consequent increase in hypothalamic GnRH release. Although GnRH is not normally detectable in the systemic circulation, it is after the menopause, indicating a considerable elevation in release. Indeed, the gonadotrophins' secretion is so enhanced that large quantities can be extracted from urine collected from post-menopausal women and used subsequently in the treatment of infertility as human post-menopausal gonadotrophin (HPG). The increase in FSH release is accompanied by a decline in inhibin secretion from the ovaries. This permits further FSH release by removal of its individual negative feedback control.

4.5 Control of the menopause

Perhaps the most difficult questions to answer are: what causes the menopause? and what determines the age at which it occurs? In Western industrialized societies, the mean menopausal age is approximately 50 years (UK 50.78 years, USA 49.8 years), but in more underdeveloped cultures, such as New Guinea, the mean age of menopause is 47.3 years. Nutrition, state of health, marital status, and tobacco smoking may all have an influence on

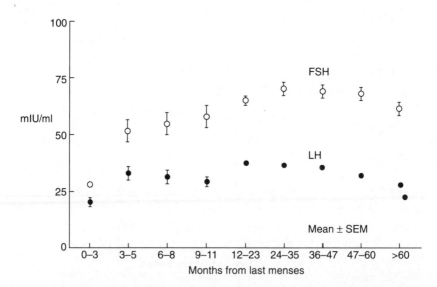

Fig. 4.6. Concentrations (mIU/ml) of FSH and LH in the group of women described in Fig. 4.4. From Longcope, C. In: Flint, M. *et al.* (1990) (ed.) *Ann. NY Acad. Sci.*, **592**, 1.

the age of onset. However, the single most important factor is the number of ovarian follicles: there appears to be a critical number of follicles at which the menopause occurs. Therefore, the timing of the phase of accelerated follicular loss (from approximately 40 to 50 years of age) and the velocity of its progress will determine when the menopause occurs. These two parameters may be determined genetically or they may be influenced by the neuroendocrine mechanisms controlling gonadotrophin secretion, since the phase of accelerated follicular loss is accompanied by rising gonadotrophin concentrations. How enhanced GnRH secretion occurs to bring about the increased gonadotrophin (LH and FSH) concentrations is not known. Reduced gonadal steroid release will, in turn, increase both GnRH and gonadotrophin secretion through the removal of the normal negative feedback exerted by oestradiol and progesterone.

As with puberty (see Chapter 3), the interactions of neurones in the mediobasal hypothalamus (MBH) which secrete dopamine, β-endorphin, and GnRH may explain the eventual increase in gonadotrophins and the irregular menstrual cycle activity. As a result of progressive changes in the MBH during middle age, the already irregular menstrual cycle activity proceeds towards complete loss of the cycles. MBH dopaminergic activity is decreased in middle age as a result of the repetitive oestrogen surges in the menstrual cycles, thus reducing dopaminergic activation of both GnRH and endorphinergic neurones. Reduced activation of the β-endorphin-secreting neurones removes the opioid inhibition of GnRH release, permitting more GnRH and gonadotrophin secretion and, hence, more oestradiol secretion. The increased oestradiol decreases dopaminergic activity in the MBH still further, leading eventually to more irregular cycles characterized by prolonged oestradiol secretion. The more oestradiol that is secreted, the more depressed is the dopaminergic activity, until eventually the menstrual cycles stop through lack of stimulation to the MBH GnRH- and β-endorphin-secreting neurones.

This explanation is based largely on work carried out on the rat oestrous cycle, which disappears in middle age. The reduced endorphinergic activity can result in a situation of opioid withdrawal, which might in part explain the hot flushes and their associated LH surges seen in women. In an animal model of opioid withdrawal, treatment of morphine-dependent rats with naloxone, an opioid antagonist, produces acute cardiac, temperature, and LH secretory changes similar in timing, magnitude, and duration to those found in the human menopause. Based on these ideas, it is possible to construct a chain of events responsible for the menopausal hot flushes. Decreased dopaminergic stimulation of the MBH combined with the very marked reduction in gonadal steroid secretion depresses the MBH endorphinergic system, which despite its very low activity, can still be activated episodically by the few remaining active dopaminergic neurones. Such episodic activation of dopaminergic neurones will stimulate GnRH secretion, thus producing the LH pulses and, at the same time, it could stimulate endorphinergic activity, producing a hyperthermic response or hot flush. How relevant these hypotheses involving neuroendocrine control of gonadotrophin secretion in the rat are to the human menopause should be the subject of considerable research in the future.

4.6 Is there a male menopause?

Since the adult human male does not show a dramatic decline in sex steroid secretion with age, it is very unlikely that a true male equivalent of the menopause exists. Some men have proved to retain their fertility into their eighties, but increasing age is accompanied by decreased bone and muscle mass, decreased pubic hair, decreased sexual activity, and decreased libido as well as decreased testicular Leydig cell mass and function. Plasma testosterone concentrations show a gradual decline from 23.55 ± 7.21 nmol/l at age 20–30 years to 15.07 ± 6.04 nmol/l at age 80–89 years. This decline is accompanied by increased plasma LH concentrations, presumably as a result of removal of some of the androgen negative feedback. Other symptoms of the reduced androgen secretion are asthenia, osteoporosis, and reduced haematocrit. At present, the cause of the decreased plasma androgen concentrations is believed to be primarily testicular in origin, due to decreased Leydig cell numbers and decreased testicular vascular perfusion. There is also evidence of altered hypothalamic–pituitary function: although the total number of LH pulses is not reduced, the frequency of high-amplitude pulses is, perhaps as a result of decreased GnRH release.

4.7 Hormone replacement therapy (HRT)

Up to 40 per cent of women develop menopausal symptoms of sufficient severity for them to seek medical advice. As these symptoms are related to the reduction in oestradiol secretion (typically symptoms begin to appear at plasma oestradiol concentrations of 35 pg/ml or lower), hormone replacement therapy (HRT) is now widely used, so the physiological consequences of this therapy should be appreciated. Early HRT preparations were oestrogen-only, containing oestradiol or long-acting analogues such as ethinyl oestradiol. Nowadays, there is a preference for a combined oestrogen and progestagen preparation, as this produces fewer side-effects. Routes of HRT have also varied. Most recently, a transdermal patch preparation has been adopted, because it delivers oestradiol at a constant level into the bloodstream. The transdermal patch system consists of a thin adhesive patch containing oestradiol in an ethanol solution; the oestradiol is delivered through a microporous membrane in close proximity to the skin surface at a constant, predictable rate for absorption, ultimately, into the systemic circulation. The site of the patch attachment does not influence absorption. Within 2–8 h of application, a maximum plasma oestradiol concentration is reached and this is sustained for up to 4 days, after which a new patch must be applied. Oral progestagen treatment is recommended between days 5 and 12 of a month's patch therapy. With this therapy, there is a reduced occurrence of hot flushes, sweating, sleep disturbances, and vaginal symptoms. Women have reported a general psychological improvement, less depression, and increased libido and sexual activity. There have also been reports of drug dependence in women receiving HRT: this could be due to direct CNS effects of the oestradiol including stimulation of endorphinergic systems in the brain.

Other side-effects of HRT have been minimal to date. There is little irritation at the site of the patch attachment and breast tenderness, abdominal bloating, nausea, breakthrough bleeding, and uterine endometrial hyperplasia have been reported. The most disturbing potential side-effect is stimulation of oestrogen-dependent cancers, such as breast and endometrial cancer, resulting from the relatively dramatic increase in plasma oestradiol concentrations. Sequential progestagen treatment, combined with the patch oestradiol delivery system, reduces all these side-effects significantly.

Patch delivery of oestradiol also reduces plasma LH and FSH concentrations, due to reactivation of the negative feedback pathways to both the anterior pituitary and hypothalamus. However, perhaps the most important effect of HRT is prevention of osteoporosis. Transdermal oestradiol increases bone mineral density in post-menopausal women with established osteoporosis by up to 6 per cent over 6–24 months. Over the same period, an untreated control group of women showed a net decline in bone mineral density of up to 4.3 per cent. Progestagens may also have a protective effect on bone. There might also be an improvement in cardiovascular function as a result of HRT. Decreased concentrations of total and LDL-cholesterol and increased concentrations of HDL-cholesterol have been reported after oestrogen-only HRT. More research is required to define the precise effects of HRT on cardiovascular function menopausally.

4.8 The menopause as a life stage

The menopause is an extremely important time during and after which dynamic changes occur not only in the reproductive system, but throughout the body. These changes are a reflection of the cessation of menstrual cycles and the decline in gonadal steroid secretion. Some symptoms resulting from the declining steroid secretion may be sufficiently severe to require hormone replacement therapy (HRT). HRT has beneficial effects in preventing and reversing osteoporosis, as well as other symptoms encountered menopausally. Oestrogen-only replacement therapy has the potential for stimulating oestrogen-dependent cancer, but combined oestrogen–progestagen therapy will overcome this particular problem. Since the actual mechanisms controlling the occurrence of the menopause are not yet understood, HRT is probably not being used as effectively as it could be. There is also a lack of knowledge, by both the general public and medical practitioners alike, of the menopause and how it influences a woman's physiology. The establishment of 'Well Woman' clinics as part of most General Medical Practices represents an important step forward. Such clinics will permit both a better assessment of the adverse symptoms associated with the menopause and their treatment.

Further reading

Balfour, J.A. and Heel, R.C. (1990). Transdermal estradiol: a review of its pharmacodynamic and pharmacokinetic properties, and therapeutic efficacy in the treatment of menopausal complaints. *Drugs*, **40**, 561–82.

Ballinger, C.B. (1990). Psychiatric aspects of the menopause. *British Journal of Psychiatry*, **156**, 773–87.

Barbo, D.M. (ed.) (1987). The postmenopausal woman. *Medical Clinics of North America*, **71**, 1–152.

Flint, M., Kronenberg, F., and Utian, W. (eds) (1990). Multi-disciplinary perspectives on menopause. *Annals of the New York Academy of Science*, **592**, 1–488.

Gambrell, R.D. Jr (ed.) (1987). The menopause. *Obstetrics and Gynecology Clinics of North America*, **14**, 1–327.

Ginsburg, J. (1991). What determines the age at the menopause? *British Medical Journal*, **302**, 1288–9.

Rasmussen, D.D. (1991). The interaction between medio-basohypothalamic dopaminergic and endorphinergic neuronal systems as a key regulator of reproduction: an hypothesis. *Journal of Endocrinological Investigation*, **14**, 323–52.

Vermeulen, A. (1991). Clinical review 24: androgens in the ageing male. *Journal of Clinical and Endocrinological Metabolism*, **73**, 221–4.

5

Old age

Summary

This chapter deals with some of the physiological changes that occur in old age. Ageing is placed in perspective and mechanisms of studying ageing, especially cellular ageing, are discussed. Thereafter an attempt is made to explain the broad concepts behind some of the multitude of hypotheses which have been suggested to account for ageing.

Finally some of the effects of ageing on different organ systems are discussed briefly. Of necessity this is not comprehensive and more specialized texts need to be consulted for details.

5.1 An ageing population

Many people are now living into their nineties and even achieving a century. Other animals, even though they have a very similar physiology, either when considered as a whole or when one considers their individual organ systems, live very different lengths of time. Mice rarely live beyond 3 years, dogs rarely exceed 20 years. Why should this be?

It is clear that a man at, for example, 80 years old, even if fit and well, is different from the same man at 20 years of age. In general he will have fewer, greyer hairs, poorer vision, poorer hearing, poorer muscle power, and poorer mobility. What are the changes that bring this about? How do we differentiate these changes from disease processes? Gerontologists are now making systematic studies of the ageing process. *Speculation* about its causes has been fashionable for hundreds of years. There has also been a continued search for a 'cure', but without success.

5.1.1 Definitions

'Ageing' and 'senescence' are terms which are frequently used without much care as to their meaning. Strictly, senescence in animal biology is the post-reproductive phase of the life span and might be very variable for males and females (see p. 122). Ageing, however, implies a decreased viability or an increased vulnerability to stress, be it internal or external; ageing has also been defined as a decreased ability to maintain homeostasis. The World Health Organization regards 45–59 as middle age, 60–74 as elderly, 75–89 as old, and 90 + as very old. Hippocrates classified ageing differently in that up to 70 is the springtime of old age, 70–75 is green old age, 75–80 is real old age, 80–90 ultimate old age, and 90 + senility. It is surprising how our perspective changes as we age!

Not all the changes that occur as an individual grows older can be regarded as strictly ageing changes. Many older people suffer debilitating diseases and there is much confusion as to what is disease and what is part of the ageing process. Perhaps it will help, to define four criteria which need to be met before a change can be regarded as ageing.

Firstly, it should be universal. This does not necessarily mean that all individuals will show the change to the same degree. Consider natural hair colour. Some individuals are completely grey at 40, while others do not show many grey hairs until they are 70 or over. Nevertheless if one waits long enough grey hairs come to all! It can therefore be regarded as an ageing change.

Secondly, the change should be intrinsic to the organism. Ultraviolet light has different effects on the physical and chemical properties of the collagen in the skin. This is brought about because of changes in the skin collagen with age. The response to the external stimulus is altered because of the internal or intrinsic change.

Thirdly, the change should be progressive and irreversible. Ideally the change should be slowly progressive and continuous and not a sudden dramatic change. In this respect occlusion of the coronary or cerebral arteries could be regarded as disease, although atheroma might arguably be regarded as an ageing process.

Finally, to be classified as ageing a change should be deleterious to the organism. This is in fact controversial. If one takes the example of the increasing cross-linkages that occur in collagen with age one is left with the problem that mature collagen is stronger than young collagen. Can this be regarded as deleterious? For most ageing changes however, there is no doubt, and reduction in muscle mass, decreased number of neurones, and a decreased cardiac performance can all be regarded as deleterious.

5.1.2 Life span

As the philosopher remarked, 'Death is the only certainty of life'. There is some uncertainty about when it will arrive however. And how should one define the life span of the population? The biblical 'three score and ten years' is now usually exceeded. Is the life span the maximum theoretical age

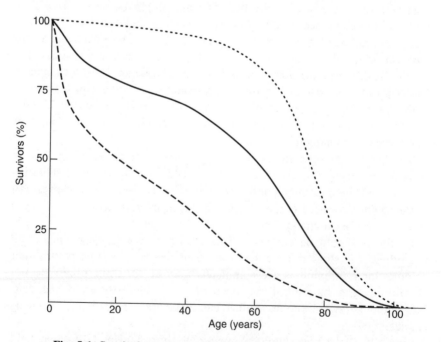

Fig. 5.1. Survival curves for different populations:
UK 1975 (------), UK 1901 (——), British India 1921–1930 (---). Survival at earlier ages has increased with the passage of time and is greater in more developed countries. Note the maximum age achieved has not altered.

to which one can live or the mean? Surprisingly when one considers different populations from different times and different countries, the maximum age achieved does not seem to have altered. When considering Fig. 5.1, however, it is easy to see that the mean age has increased in developed countries with time and is greater in developed than in underdeveloped countries. All the advances in medicine have not succeeded in extending the theoretical life span, they have just helped more people to nearly achieve it.

For the purposes of insuring life the commercial companies have developed tables from which it can be predicted what chance there is of a person of any given age dying. Gerontologists are also interested in such relationships because age–mortality relationships may show whether ageing changes (as opposed to pathological changes) are occurring in the population. If, as discussed above, ageing does imply an increased vulnerability to external or internal stresses that may result in death, there will be a progressive increase in the age-specific death rate. This can be defined as the proportion of people who die in a specified time interval when compared with those who were alive at its beginning. This is sometimes called the force of mortality. The increase in age-specific death rates was shown to be exponential many years ago by the English actuary Gompertz. It can be expressed mathematically as

$$R_t = R_0 e^{\alpha t}$$

where R_t is the mortality at age t, R_0 is the hypothetical mortality at the age of maturity (which Gompertz took as 35 years) and α is the rate at which the force of mortality increases in the ageing population—sometimes called the Gompertz coefficient (see Fig. 5.2).

5.1.3 Increasing the life span

The maximum life span for humans seems to be approximately 100–110 years but there are still relatively few people living in the UK who exceed 100 years. The ratio of women to men at 100 is approximately 6:1 and even at 75 women outnumber men by 2:1.

Documentary evidence of extreme longevity is hard to come by though there are many unsubstantiated stories. The Amerindians of the Ecuadorian Andes are reputed to live to great ages with 142 years being reported. The Abkhasians of Russia and the Hunzas who live on the borders of Bangladesh and China are also tribes with reputed longevity. However, care must be taken in assessing such claims. Sometimes documentary evidence can be 'modified', for example, to escape military service and the practice in some areas of sons adopting their fathers' names makes for great confusion. All the groups where extreme longevity is reported have some common features: there is a low density of population, there is a frugal diet with little animal protein, the family groups are close knit, and they all have the active physical life associated with an agricultural economy. Whether any of these factors is significant in influencing longevity is not known. Amerindians consume on average two to four cups of unrefined rum and 40–60 cigarettes per day. This just highlights the difficulty in trying to assess factors which increase life span.

Many factors that increase longevity are genetically determined and it is essential, if one wants to achieve long life, to choose one's parents carefully. For some reason the age of one's mother at conception does seem to have a

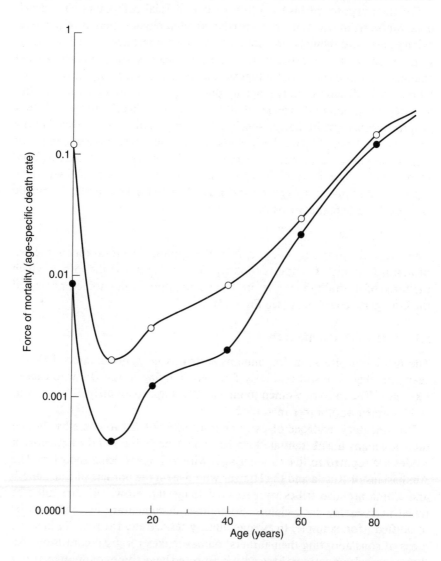

Fig. 5.2. Gompertz plot of force of mortality for English males in 1910 (—○—) and 1960 (— ●—). The Gompertz coefficient (α) applies in this graph to ages over 40. Based on figures from the Registrar General's Decennial Supplement (1961).

statistical relationship with longevity. Offspring born early in a mother's reproductive life tend to live longer than those born at the end. More careful work has been done with animal populations. Selective breeding for long-lived mutants of the nematode *Caenorhabditis elegans* has produced an increase in life span of 67 per cent. Several different genes appear to be involved and their identification may give important clues to ageing.

Several environmental factors have also been tested in animals. Growth retardation, which has been produced by caloric restriction, has been shown to be important in nematodes and rats. The effects on rats are complicated in that caloric restriction before weaning shortens life span but caloric restriction in the immediate post-weaning period extends life span; restrictions later in life have no apparent effects. One observation that has caused intense speculation is that in the fruit fly *Drosophila melanogaster* an increased frequency of sexual intercourse has deleterious effects on life span; there is no evidence that this applies to humans.

5.1.4 Effect of ageing on population structure

Animals in the wild rarely show signs of great age because when an animal begins to fail, it is either left to die or killed by predators or sometimes even the same herd. Humans frequently behave differently and because of the improvements in medical care the number of old people in the population is growing. In the UK at present there are 10 million people over 65 years of age; all the predictions are that this will increase until by the year 2000 the number of 60 year olds will have increased by 50 per cent and there will be 3.5 million people over 75. Gerontology studies are therefore not only desirable but mandatory. As the population grows older some 20–25 per cent of the population will be showing significant ageing changes. This will pose the major problem for health and social services in the future.

5.2 Studies of ageing

5.2.1 Man

In man there are simple yet cogent reasons why ageing studies are difficult to perform. To avoid dramatic changes in external influences such as the changing quality of medical care, public health, and hygiene it is necessary to use longitudinal studies where a cohort of individuals can be followed throughout their lives. This would involve a team working for over 100 years to follow all the cohort from cradle to grave!

Cross-sectional studies are more practical but raise problems with interpretation because different external influences may have influenced the groups. For example, 60 year olds of the present time (1994) had a restricted diet during their childhood years because of rationing during the Second World War. Forty year olds never suffered the same privations. Will this account for some of the changes seen when they are studied and so be wrongly attributed to ageing? Members of older groups are specially selected in that they have survived all the rigours of life and so may not be typical of their cohort.

5.2.2 Animals

Since senescence is rare in wild populations, animal studies are, in some respects, more difficult than those in man. Some species, such as the albatross, mountain sheep, Arctic fin whale, and tortoise undoubtedly live to a great age but many experiments on survival depend on records from zoos and are not really representative of what happens in nature.

5.2.3 Cells

So far we have considered ageing as a process applying to the body as a whole. We really need to ask the question, 'Does ageing occur in cells?', because if so, perhaps they can be studied in isolation.

In the body there are basically three types of cells:

(1) highly specialized ones which have lost the ability to reproduce;
(2) highly specialized cells that are capable of division but usually do not do so frequently; and
(3) less specialized cells that readily undergo division.

These latter two types of cells can be grown in culture.

Over 60 years ago it was shown that cultured chick heart muscle cells divided so many times that the life span of the tissue culture greatly exceeded the life span of the animal from which those cells were derived. It was even postulated that the cells were immortal. However, it seems likely that new generations of cells were inadvertently transferred to these cultures with the nutrient media.

So far, many cells which appear to be immortal have been shown to be abnormal in their chromosomal make-up. One of the earliest cell lines, the HeLa cell (derived from a cervical carcinoma from Helen Lane) has been cultured for more than 30 years but each cell now has between 50 and 300 chromosomes. Stem cells from germ or haematopoetic cell lines, however, may be regarded as immortal.

Human fibroblasts are the most widely studied cell model of ageing. Over 25 years ago Hayflick showed that fibroblasts had a limited life span in culture. Fetal lung fibroblasts propagated for 60 divisions and then stopped. The number of divisions seems to be critical rather than the time in culture. Cells which are artificially stopped from dividing (by manipulation of the culture media) after 30 divisions, if started again will only divide a further 30 times.

Table 5.1. Life span of fibroblasts*

Species	Number of times population of fibroblasts in culture doubles	Maximum life span (years)
Galapagos tortoise	90–125	175 (?)
Man	40–60	110
Mink	30–34	10
Chicken	15–35	30
Mouse	14–28	3.5

* From Hayflick, L. (1975). *Federation Proceedings*, **34**, 9–13.

5.2.4 Relationship between cellular ageing and ageing of the organism

The relationship between ageing changes *in vivo* and *in vitro* is still hotly debated. There seems to be a crude relationship between the number of times a fibroblast can divide and the life span of the animal from which it is derived (Table 5.1) but this may not be so for all cell types. In addition, the maximum number of times a human fibroblast will divide is correlated inversely with the age of the donor, although cells from a centagenarian can still divide approximately 40 times compared with 60 for fetal cells. Interestingly in diseases such as progeria or Werner's syndrome where there is premature ageing, the fibroblasts have a reduced number of divisions in culture.

Ageing fibroblasts show biochemical and morphological changes reminiscent of ageing changes *in vivo*. For example, there are increased numbers of larger lysosomes, increased numbers of chromosomal abnormalities, and the rates of translation, transcription, and protein degradation are usually reduced. In general old fibroblasts *in vivo* and *in vitro* show reduced sensitivity to growth factors and hormones and they may accumulate structurally altered protein.

Interestingly, if old fibroblasts are fused with young phenotypes the hybrids show inhibition of the synthesis of DNA in the nucleus. Old cells seem to contain abundant mRNA for short-lived membrane proteins which cause this inhibition. It is possible that there is an age-related increase in some inhibitor of cell cycle progression, possibly an oncogene, a phosphatase, or a protease.

5.3 Theories of ageing

If we really understood more about ageing there would be fewer hypotheses about its cause. Some 300 hypotheses refer to ageing of cells or ageing of the organism. A lot of effort has been expended trying to reach a unifying theory of ageing, but whether this is useful is doubtful, since there seem to be many concurrent changes. The following theories have been grouped to avoid giving details of all.

5.3.1 Hypotheses of cellular ageing

These hypotheses assume that there is a time-dependent degradation of cellular information. If this leads to death of the cell, it can become very significant if similar cells cannot reproduce to make good the loss (see p. 112). It might be of course that the hypotheses are not mutually exclusive. In general they can be divided into error theories or programme theories.

5.3.1.1 *Error theories*

In general these theories postulate some error or damage in cells which either gets passed on or is so catastrophic that the cells die immediately.

A group of theories postulates that there is some alteration in the information carried by the DNA and that this error is passed on to the next generation. Damage could be from mutations or more likely from breaking or cross-linking of the DNA strands which would inevitably increase with the number of replications that occur. It may be that damage to DNA is much commoner than previously thought and the error is in the repair mechanisms which normally limit the damage.

A widely tested theory was proposed more than 30 years ago and depended on two facts:

(1) that transfer of information from DNA to RNA is not perfect; and

(2) that proteins themselves are involved with this information transfer.

A low level of synthesis of aberrant proteins was proposed to lead eventually to catastrophic production of malfunctioning proteins since a number of proteins such as RNA polymerase, tRNA synthetases, and ribosomal proteins would all work to produce abnormal proteins in their turn. Although early work in *Neurospora* supported this, it now seems unlikely since old cells synthesize proteins as faithfully as young cells. It is true that there are increased levels of aberrant proteins but these probably arise from post-translational modifications rather than errors in translation of the message of DNA.

There are several protein modifications which increase with age and accumulate within cells. Non-enzymatic glycosylation and alteration of cross-linkages of macromolecules have been shown to occur in a variety of cells (see Table 5.2). There may also be changes in protein degradation. Catabolism of long-lived proteins declines in old human fibroblasts and in many cells there is a reduction of lysosomal proteolysis.

Free radicals are chemical species that contain an unpaired electron in an outer orbital which makes them very reactive. They can attack DNA or

Table 5.2. Examples of some protein alterations which accumulate in ageing cells

Protein	Modification with age	Tissue
Aldolase	Proteolytic fragments	Mouse liver
Band 3 protein	Oxidation, proteolytic fragments	Human red cells
Maltase	Conformational changes	Rat kidney
Collagen	Oxidation, non-enzymatic glycosylation	Human tendon
Triose-phosphate isomerase	Deamidation of asparagine residues	Human {lymphocytes {fibroblasts

proteins but a major effect may be to cause peroxidation of membrane lipids. When they damage molecules they also tend to produce more free radicals. The number of molecules showing oxidative damage has been shown to increase in ageing platelets and endothelial cells in culture.

Lipofuscin is a pigment derived from non-enzymatic glycosylation of structural proteins and DNA. After glycosylation the sugar groups can be oxidized to form massive cross-links between proteins, lipids, and nucleic acids and some of the conjugates fluoresce. It is not known whether accumulation of lipofuscin is itself damaging or is merely a consequence of a more fundamental problem. Inhibitors of lysosomal enzymes can lead to a premature accumulation of lipofuscin in the brain and liver but whether this accelerates ageing is not yet clear.

5.3.1.2 *Programme theories*

There is no doubt that some cells are programmed to die. The reabsorption of a tadpole's tail, the death of eclosal muscles used during insect metamorphosis, and death of cells between the digits in developing mammals are all examples of apoptosis (programmed cell death) but whether this is the mechanism by which most cells die is not known.

Some genes are repeated many times in cells. It has been suggested that selective damage to one of these repetitive genes will result in activation of another copy. When the last copy has been used, if the gene product is important then the cells die. It must be admitted, however, that many proteins are encoded by a single gene and so this is not likely to be a general mechanism.

When cells replicate their chromosomes prior to cell division, it has been proposed that the last parts of the DNA sequences to replicate may be lost. If one assumes (and it is a big assumption) that non-essential DNA sequences are at the ends of the replicating units, these would gradually be reduced until an essential gene was lost and the cell died. Recently a variant of the theory has been proposed. Telomeres are repeats of hexanucleide sequences at the ends of chromosomes; in humans, for example, the sequence TTAGGG is repeated until it reaches a length of 4 kb. This is added to the ends of chromosomes after replication. Maybe some telomeres are lost after each replication eventually causing damage to vital genes. In support of this idea it has been noted that when fibroblasts grow old in culture the mean size of the telomere is only 2 kb; and cells from patients with premature ageing (progeria) also have short telomere sequences. Confirmatory data have been obtained from yeast cells. Of course rather than a programmed event, the same effect could be produced by an error in the telomerase enzyme which adds on the telomeres.

A further set of theories envisage that after a certain number of cell divisions a particular gene (or genes) may be switched on. Ageing fibroblasts preferentially express a number of genes which may or may not inhibit the progress of a cell through its cycle before division. A potent inhibitor of cell growth for endothelial cells is interleukin-1α (IL-1α) which can act in a paracrine fashion. Interestingly, when endogenous production of IL-1α is inhibited, the maximum number of divisions that occurs in cultured cells increases from 60 to 140. There are also reductions in a number of stimulators of cell division in cultured cells such as the c-*fos* gene, whose expression is essential for DNA synthesis. In old cells its transcription is reduced. However, it seems unlikely that a single gene effect could account for ageing since at least 13 cell regulatory proteins are poorly expressed in old cells while five are unaltered.

It is probable that ageing is a multifactorial process and that single defects cannot account for the changes.

5.3.2 Ageing of the whole organism

While not denying theories of cellular ageing, this set of hypotheses concentrates on changes in whole tissue or changes widely disseminated throughout the body.

5.3.2.1 *Wear and tear*

There have been many suggestions that ageing is simply due to wearing out of body parts which are non-replaceable. It is fairly obvious that when carnivores lose their teeth, they can no longer feed and so age and die. Similarly as neurones wear out or are damaged, cardiac muscle cells cease to function, and nephrons are lost in the kidney so the body is less able to respond to changes. Effectively the functional reserve is reduced. When this functional reserve disappears, the organism can no longer maintain homeostasis and ageing and death follow.

Steady loss of irreplaceable substances is a variant of these hypotheses. Such exhaustion undoubtedly occurs but its importance in causing ageing is not certain. Loss of elastin from skin, arteries, and lens is obviously one classical example of non-replacement of a substance in a variety of organs. There is a strong correlation between metabolic rate and ageing in different animal species and even within the same species. For example, if the metabolic rate of cold blooded animals is reduced, the animals live longer.

It could be objected however that wear and tear is a result of rather than the cause of ageing.

5.3.2.2 *Excess accumulation*

Accumulation of substances in abnormal or inappropriate places has been suggested as a cause for ageing. While accumulation of lipofuscin has already been mentioned (see p. 109), other substances may be important. Collagen is laid down between myocardial cells, amyloid is laid down in brain plaques, and calcium may be found in the media or subendothelial layer of large arteries. These latter changes may predispose to lipid deposits. Again, however, many of these changes may be a consequence of rather than a primary cause of ageing.

5.3.2.3 *Endocrine changes*

Hormones are important in homeostasis and homeostatic mechanisms are disturbed in ageing. Perhaps hormone loss can cause ageing changes. While some changes in the ageing process can be reversed by hormone supplementation—witness the striking results of hormone replacement therapy in some post-menopausal women (see Chapter 4)—the general pattern of ageing cannot.

Plasma concentrations of thyroxine, cortisol, growth hormone, ACTH, and TSH do not change significantly with age. Changes in pituitary gonadotrophins increase because there is a loss of the normal negative feedback mechanism. While some changes occur because of this, there is no evidence for a primary role in ageing. Measuring plasma concentrations of hormones may not tell the whole story since, while plasma concentrations may not alter, there is sometimes a change in the sensitivity of receptors. For example, while plasma insulin concentrations are not reduced in older people, the response to insulin is diminished because of decreased receptor density.

A development of these theories is the concept of a neuroendocrine clock (which is entirely different from that involved in the circadian rhythmicity described in Chapter 10). The neuroendocrine clock would control neurotransmitters and hormones which could cause homeostatic changes throughout the body. It might even ultimately control transcription and translational processes through hormones. If such a clock does exist and the evidence for it is meagre, then perhaps ageing could be controlled by biofeedback techniques. 'You're only as old as you feel', could then become a reality rather than an anodyne.

5.3.2.4 *Ageing and the immune system*

These hypotheses bridge the cellular and overall theories of ageing. Damage to lymphocytes might cause the manufacture of abnormal antibodies perhaps even against the individual's own tissues. Alternatively manifestation of abnormal proteins on cell surfaces could stimulate antibody production and cells would no longer be recognized as belonging to that individual. In either case ageing would be viewed as an autoimmune disease. Some diseases associated with ageing are related to immunological disorders; these include Type II diabetes mellitus, giant cell arteritis, and amyloidosis. Tests that depend on a competent immune system, such as the Mantoux test for tuberculosis, become negative in elderly patients. Immunological surveillance may also become imapired with age so that abnormal cells, which are normally destroyed, no longer are.

5.3.3 Summary of causes

It can be seen from the foregoing, which itself is only a summary, that there is no consensus on the cause of ageing. Life can be viewed as a series of interacting systems of unstable chemicals; with the passage of time they may just be reduced to their lowest energy state and no longer be reactive—this would be death. Changes in the body occur simultaneously at many different sites and the theories of ageing are not mutually exclusive. The search continues for the primary cause.

5.4 Effects of ageing

Age changes occur in most systems of the body. Where there is no replacement of dead cells (brain, muscle, and heart) these changes are manifest early and dramatically; where continual replacement occurs (red cells and intestinal epithelium) the changes may be minimal or not easily noticed. In general, complex functions involving co-ordination are affected much more than simple ones. For example, reaction time to respond to a stimulus is slowed much more than conduction velocity in the nerves. In Fig. 5.3 a selection of changes are presented. These demonstrate how widespread the effects are. It is possible in some respects to group changes from different systems. For example, loss of elastic tissue affects the skin, cardiovascular system, lungs, and lens of the eye. This enables us to identify some unifying themes.

There is a fine distinction between diseases *associated with* old age and changes which are *due* to old age. The changes presented below are ageing changes that occur, to a greater or lesser extent, in all old people. We will not discuss the myriad of diseases which afflict some of the elderly.

5.4.1 The nervous system

5.4.1.1 *Neuroanatomical changes*

Brain weight may decrease by 6–7 per cent between 20 and 80 years of age. The surface area of the cerebral cortex is decreased and there is a general-

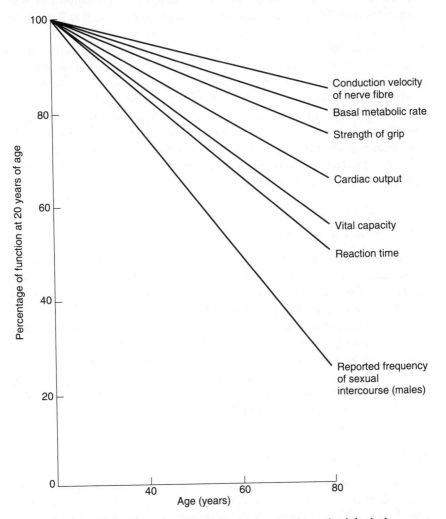

Fig. 5.3. Diagram showing deterioration of various physiological functions as a percentage of that function at 20 years of age. Data from Bromley, D.B. (1974). *The psychology of human ageing*, 2nd edn, p. 93, Pelican Books.

ized smoothing of the various sulci and gyri. Although it is frequently stated that brain cells are lost at a rate of approximately 10 000 per day from age 20 onwards the evidence for this is not good and is based on cross-sectional studies (see p. 105) of post-mortem tissue. In addition, careful work has shown that as neurones are lost the dendrites of the remainder become longer and form more connections, thus compensating to some extent. Some of the loss may be secondarily related to impaired blood supply.

The relationship of ageing with Alzheimer's disease is complex and not fully understood. Alzheimer's disease is characterized by amyloid deposition around neurofibrillary tangles and while these can occur anywhere they seem to predominate in the hippocampus and limbic systems. Sometimes these findings can be demonstrated at post-mortem although the patient showed no evidence of symptoms. They only occur in a small section of the population. Post-mortem examination in many people reveals amyloid deposition in the brain; this does seem to increase with age as do the neuritic plaques which are composed of degenerating neuronal processes, amyloid material, and invading neuroglial cells. While these latter probably satisfy all the criteria (see p. 101) for an ageing process, Alzheimer's disease probably does not since there is considerable dispute about its universality.

Lipofuscin (see p. 109) is accumulated by many nerve cells, but its relation to the cause of ageing is not known.

5.4.1.2 *Neurochemical changes*

Depletion of neurotransmitters generally occurs with age. A decrease of dopamine occurs in the substantia nigra of the basal ganglia and when this progresses far enough will lead to Parkinsonian-like symptoms. Some forms of tremor associated with old age may be related to this.

Other neurotransmitters are also depleted. Loss of noradrenaline and 5-hydroxytryptamine in the hypothalamus may be associated with depression; low concentrations of homovanillic acid (a metabolite of monoamines) and of acetylcholine in the hypothalamus may be associated with senile dementia. The cause of senile dementia, however, is probably multifactorial and the role of transmitters is unclear.

5.4.1.3 *Higher nervous function*

We have little knowledge about the physiology of higher nervous function although there is much conjecture. It is not surprising then that ageing changes are not understood. Mental confusion is very frequent in the elderly and old people have difficulty in orientating themselves in time and space. Whether this is a result of disease processes or is specifically an ageing change is not known.

Short-term memory is one function which has been well studied. Long-term memory is surprisingly well preserved but short-term memory is impaired, sometimes severely. This may be linked to a decreased ability to learn new skills in old age. Complex functions such as conceptual skills and reasoning ability begin to decline very early but verbal skills are relatively well preserved. Frequently, elderly people, by making use of experience, can mask this loss of intellectual capacity.

Sleep and its quality are changed with age. The amount of REM sleep progressively reduces with age and sleep patterns are disturbed. Sometimes this is caused by nocturia but even when this does not occur elderly people sleep less at night and nap during the day. The total time spent 'unconscious' may not vary much.

5.4.1.4 *Regulatory function*

Many of the body's regulatory mechanisms are impaired in later life. One mechanism commonly affected is postural control and this is often noted in the shuffling gait and stooping posture of the elderly. If an elderly person stumbles or is pushed and the centre of gravity is displaced, they are less able to correct, partly because of slow reflexes and partly because the weakened muscles do not have the same speed or strength of response. As a result many falls occur and these can cause tremendous problems.

Autonomic regulation also suffers with age. Bladder and bowel function, especially sphincter control, is impaired and incontinence results. Autonomic control of blood pressure (see p. 118) and body temperature (see p. 116) are also disturbed with age.

5.4.1.5 *The peripheral nervous system*

Peripheral nerves are affected less than central ones. The maximum speed of nerve conduction (see Fig. 5.3) decreases slightly with age and the speed of simple reflexes is slightly less but in general peripheral function is preserved. There is some loss of motoneurones from the spinal cord.

5.4.2 Special senses

As age progresses hearing and sight are both impaired and this may eventually lead to deafness or blindness.

5.4.2.1 *Vision*

The arcus senilis is a white border around the cornea caused by fatty infiltration. While this seems to be an invariable concomitant of old age there is no known functional significance.

Much more serious changes occur in the lens. Because it is composed of elastic tissues within an elastic envelope the lens suffers as do all elastic tissues in the body from replacement of elastin by more rigid molecules. As a result the lens is less able to change its shape and becomes stiffer, reducing the ability of the eye to accommodate for near vision. The near point recedes and this becomes obvious from approximately 40–50 years of age. The water content of the lens tissue critically determines its transparent nature. Changes in hydration of the lens fibres will give rise to opacities and senile cataracts and these increase as age progresses.

Changes also occur in the retina. Blood vessels grow into the retina from the choroid and may become leaky, giving rise to haemorrhages or exudates. If these occur in younger people the debris is removed by pigmented epithelial cells but with age this mechanism deteriorates. Rods and cones around the exudates die off eventually. Small opaque bodies occur in the vitreous humour and are noticed because black dots float across the visual field. In general visual acuity is reduced with age.

Cataracts, glaucoma, and retinopathy due to diabetes mellitus or hypertension are much commoner among elderly people but are not truly changes due to ageing.

5.4.2.2 *Hearing*

Many problems arise with hearing in old age, ranging from excessive wax production in the external auditory meatus (which gives rise to conduction deafness) to loss of hair cells on the basilar membrane. Loss of elasticity of the tympanic and basilar membranes of the cochlear impair hearing and most older people suffer from presbyacusis—the loss of the ability to recognize higher frequency tones—which may be associated with hypersensitivity to loud noises. Tinnitus and impairment of sound localization are increasingly frequent with old age but their cause is not clear.

5.4.2.3 *Chemical senses*

Taste is impaired in elderly people partly because of a loss of taste buds and partly due to reduced saliva production. Use of dentures in many older people also impairs taste. The associated loss of smell is a contributory factor. Smell is probably impaired because of degeneration of neurones in the olfactory bulb.

5.4.3 Temperature regulation

For a variety of reasons temperature regulation is not as good in elderly people. This arises partly because of problems with temperature appreciation and partly because of impaired mechanisms for generation of heat.

Poor control of the cardiovascular reflexes means changes in skin blood flow cannot be as easily controlled. The control mechanisms in the hypothalamus are less able to cope with a fall in temperature (which is the major problem) and older people are less aware of the temperature of the surroundings. There is increased loss of heat from thinning skin which has less subcutaneous fat; bald heads especially lose a tremendous amount of heat. Because of a number of social factors poor heating of houses and sometimes inadequate clothing contribute to the problem.

In addition, the elderly have problems generating extra heat. Vigorous exercise is not usually an option for heat production and even shivering seems to be reduced. There is a general decrease in metabolic processes; in a series of patients who had recovered from accidental hypothermia it was shown that they had no increased oxygen consumption in response to cooling.

Surprisingly in a study of old people in London a deep body temperature of less than 35.5°C occurred in at least 10 per cent of those observed, with an even lower temperature in the morning.

5.4.4 The cardiovascular and respiratory systems

While there are some changes in metabolism the fall in basal metabolic rate and oxygen consumption/unit body weight which is seen in the elderly is mainly a consequence of the reduced muscle mass and increased fat content of the body. Thus, reduced demands are placed on the delivery of oxygen during old age.

In general, the changes in the cardiovascular system can be attributed to a decline in controlling mechanisms (perhaps because of loss of nerve cells), loss of some muscle cells, and a decrease in their strength and speed of contraction. Heart rate does not significantly alter with age if measured at rest, but the maximum heart rate that can be achieved (with any stimulus) decreases from approximately 200 to 160 beats/min and this is not improved with training. The intrinsic rate of the heart (that is, when there is no vagal or sympathetic drive to the heart) is also reduced with age. In general there is a gradual loss of pacemaker cells with fibrous infiltration in the sinuatrial node which may be partly responsible for the arrhythmias which occur in up to 80 per cent of the elderly at some time. Most of the arrhythmias are supraventricular or ventricular ectopic beats. The change of heart rate with respiratory movements, sinus arrhythmia, is lost with age. The atrioventricular node is well preserved histologically, although there is an increase in PR interval on the ECG and the bundle of His is intact. There may be some loss of Purkinje fibres, especially those to the left ventricle.

The stroke volume at rest may not be different in the elderly, but it is associated with an increased left ventricle volume which can be seen radiographically as an increase in the ventricular luminal diameter during diastole.

This indicates a shift to the right of the pressure–volume curve. As a result of the increases in chamber volume the heart appears larger on X-ray examination. The maximum stroke volume that can be achieved is reduced. As a result of the changes in heart rate and stroke volume it should be obvious that while cardiac output at rest may be normal or decline slightly because of a reduced body mass, the maximum increase in cardiac output is restricted.

These changes may reflect the increase in connective tissue in the ageing heart, which shows fragmentation of elastin and its replacement by collagen. As a result the compliance of the heart is lower, that is, it has to work harder to expel the same volume of blood. There are scattered deposits of amyloid material and lipofuscin within and between cells. Valvular thickening and calcium deposits also impair functioning of heart valves, decreasing the efficiency of the heart.

A marked decrease in the response to β-adrenergic stimulation has been noted so intrinsically and extrinsically the heart is less able to respond to any challenge.

Mean blood pressure rises in the elderly. Since cardiac output is normal the increase in systolic blood pressure can be attributed to a decreased aortic compliance and loss of elasticity. The increase in diastolic pressure indicates an increased peripheral resistance. It is difficult to decide when the increased blood pressure becomes abnormal. Some would set the maximum normal blood pressure as low as 160 mm Hg systolic and 90 mm Hg diastolic although this is debatable. What is apparent from cohort studies is that over age 75–80 there is a decrease in diastolic blood pressure. There are also differences between the rise in blood pressure between the sexes. While in general systolic and diastolic pressures are lower in females than males between 20 and 30, the rise in females is steeper and after 60–65 females have higher systolic blood pressure than men (see Fig. 5.4). Control of blood pressure through the baroreceptor mechanisms is impaired in both sexes and this can cause severe postural hypotension. Many falls in the elderly can be attributed to rising suddenly from a sitting or recumbent position.

Breathing is disturbed in the elderly mainly due to loss of elastic tissue in the lungs—this decreases compliance and increases the work of breathing. There is a decrease in vital capacity together with an increase in residual volume. While none of these interfere with function at rest the ability to increase the oxygen delivery to tissues is markedly decreased. In general alveolar function is normal.

5.4.5 The kidney and body fluids

The kidney is affected by the general changes which occur in the vascular system. Sclerosis of the vessels in the glomeruli increases with age and affects 30–40 per cent of the nephrons by the age of 80. There may be frank ischaemia in parts of the kidney. Generally the glomerular basement membrane is thickened but measurements of its permeability have not been made, at least in humans.

As a consequence of these changes there is a profound fall in renal plasma flow and glomerular filtration rate, so much so that after 80 years they may only be approximately 50 per cent of their values at 30. In general they decline by approximately 10 per cent per decade. Tubular function of the

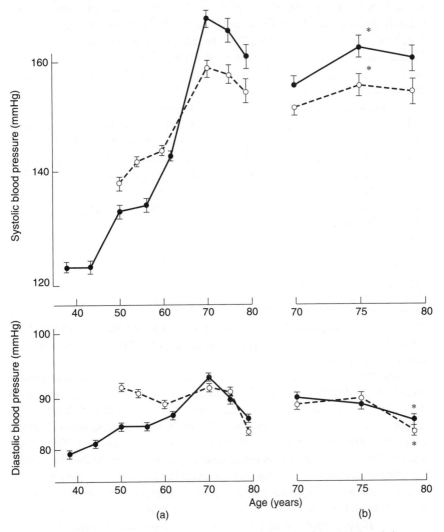

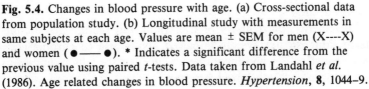

Fig. 5.4. Changes in blood pressure with age. (a) Cross-sectional data from population study. (b) Longitudinal study with measurements in same subjects at each age. Values are mean ± SEM for men (X----X) and women (●——●). * Indicates a significant difference from the previous value using paired *t*-tests. Data taken from Landahl *et al.* (1986). Age related changes in blood pressure. *Hypertension*, **8**, 1044–9.

remaining nephrons seems to be reasonably well preserved and there is even an increase in reabsorptive capacity for glucose, so that elderly diabetics may not show glycosuria.

The major problem, however, is that the functional reserve of the kidney is reduced and it is less able to compensate for disturbing influences. For example, the ability to cope with sodium depletion and sodium loading are both impaired. Whether this is due to a functional change in the nephron or to changes in controlling hormones is not known. Renal concentrating and diluting abilities are both disturbed. Studies in humans indicate that this may be due to impaired transport in the thick limb of the ascending loop of Henle; studies in rats, however, suggest there is impaired responsiveness of collecting duct cells to arginine vasopressin. Usually in the elderly there is an increased incidence of volume depletion and hypernatraemia and this may be compounded by a decrease in thirst mechanisms.

There are also problems for the elderly in excreting an acid or alkaline load. Calcium metabolism is significantly altered, although this probably relates more to decreased intestinal absorption than to altered renal tubular function. Secretory mechanisms in the kidney are impaired. This is particularly important when one considers the drugs normally excreted by the kidney; there is thus a danger of producing toxicity unless plasma levels are carefully monitored.

5.4.6 The gastrointestinal tract

With modern dentistry it might be argued that loss of teeth should not be part of the ageing process, but usually it is the most obvious gastrointestinal manifestation of age. There is consequent restructuring of the mandible and alteration of facial features.

Many old people have difficulties with swallowing. This is predominantly due to reduced saliva production but ageing changes in the brainstem nuclei may also have a role. Hiatus hernia, where part of the stomach enters the thorax, is a frequent occurrence in the elderly but its cause is not known. Since it is seen in approximately 70 per cent of people over 70 it could reasonably be ascribed to ageing. Secretion of gastric juice decreases with age and achlorhydria, with loss of intrinsic factor secretion, may develop. The villi of the small bowel mucosa become shorter and broader reducing the area available for absorption and some degree of malabsorption, particularly of folic acid, vitamin B_{12}, calcium, iron, and vitamin D almost always occurs.

Movements, particularly of the colon and rectum are diminished and defecation can be severely impaired giving rise to chronic constipation. With constipation and incontinence one can see why many elderly people are preoccupied with bowel function.

5.4.7 Skin and hair

Because of loss of elasticity of the skin, the number of wrinkles increases with age. These are accentuated by the loss of subcutaneous fat. Skin becomes thinner and more vulnerable to minor trauma causing multiple bruising (senile purpura). Pressure sores may develop but are usually secondary to diseases causing immobility. In the normal elderly they should not occur.

Hair loss with age is invariable. Everyone is familiar with male pattern baldness which is linked to androgen secretion, but even females suffer thinning of hair on the head. Axillary and pubic hair share in the general thinning but there is extra growth of coarse hairs in the nostrils and ears. In females there is an increased tendency for hair production on the upper lip.

Hair also changes its colour. There is much variation in the time at which this occurs but eventually all hair goes grey. This is due to the failure of tyrosinase, the enzyme which is responsible for pigment formation in hair.

5.4.8 The musculoskeletal system

5.4.8.1 *Bone and joints*

After the age of 45–50 the amount of bone in the body decreases. In the shaft of long bones there is an increase in both internal and external diameters. Calcification of the remaining bone is usually normal but there is a loss of bone matrix known as osteoporosis. This loss is enhanced in post-menopausal women by lack of oestrogen. Immobility also plays a role since bone is normally being constantly remodelled in response to the stresses to which it is exposed. The weakened bone predisposes to fractures and may contribute to the general 'aches and pains' to which the elderly are prone.

Joints are all subject to wear and tear which is most obvious in the weight bearing joints of the lower limb. As a person ages so the articular cartilage of the joint wears thin and may ultimately be destroyed, with bony outgrowths (osteophytes) developing at the edge of the articular surface. The osteophytes themselves may cause symptoms by pressure on neighbouring structures or they may break off and get trapped in the joint. Some degree of osteoarthritis is present in everyone after the age of 50 and this is especially noticeable in radiographs of the spine. In many cases, however, this gives rise to no symptoms.

5.4.8.2 *Intervertebral discs*

The water content of the fibrocartilaginous intervertebral discs decreases with age. As age progresses the hard outer rim of the disc (the annulus fibrosus) may become cracked and either allow the gelatinous centre (the nucleus pulposus) to protrude or itself become displaced. Either way, pressure on the spinal nerve roots ensues and gives rise to lumbago, sciatica, and a host of other ill-defined back problems. These are almost invariably found in the elderly.

5.4.8.3 *Muscle*

Although muscle structure does not seem to vary with age the total mass does and this accounts for the fall in lean body mass which is characteristic of ageing. The cause of the reduction is partly disuse atrophy—in general muscles are less used in the elderly although this can be mitigated by training—and partly due to loss of motorneurones supplying the muscle. Decreased blood supply and decreased secretion of anabolic steroids may both contribute to the process.

5.4.9 The reproductive system

There are dramatic changes in reproductive function in females (see Chapter 4). The ovarian response fails after the menopause, which usually occurs at 45–55 years although there is wide variation. This leads to a decrease in plasma concentration of oestrogen and progesterone, their negative feedback is lost, and, consequently, there is a rise in follicle-stimulating hormone and luteinizing hormone. Because of the hormonal changes there is involution of the uterus, thinning of the vaginal epithelium, and diminution of vaginal and cervical secretions. The vulva atrophies and both mammary and adipose tissue in the breasts is reduced.

In males the changes are less dramatic and more gradual. There is a reduction in testicular size and a thickening of the basement membrane which supports the germinal epithelium. Spermatozoa may be produced well into old age. Anecdotal stories outnumber hard facts but there is good documentary evidence that some men retain their sexual potency into their nineties. Hormonal secretion from the testis is reduced and there is considerable loss of libido (although this may reflect an increase in truthfulness!) (see Fig. 5.3).

Another significant change which seems to occur in all males is enlargement of the prostate, particularly the anterior lobe. This has marked effects on bladder emptying and may account for some of the nocturia seen in males.

Further reading

Brocklehurst, J.C. (ed.) (1985). *Textbook of geriatric medicine and gerontology*, 3rd edn. Churchill Livingstone, Edinburgh.
Brocklehurst, J.C. and Allen, S.C. (1987). *Geriatric medicine for students*. Churchill Livingstone, Edinburgh.

Davies, I. (1983). *Ageing. Outline studies in biology*, No. 151. Edward Arnold, London.

Dice, J.F. (1993). Cellular and molecular mechanisms of ageing. *Physiological Reviews*, **73**, 149–60.

Sinclair, D. (1985). *Human growth after birth*, 4th edn. Oxford Medical Publications, Oxford.

Svanborg, A. and Folkow, B. (1993). Physiology of cardiovascular ageing. *Physiological Reviews*, **73**, 725–64.

6

Altered temperature

6.1 Introduction

Like other mammals, humans are homeothermic animals. We normally keep our core temperature within the narrow range of 36–38°C despite large fluctuations in the environmental temperature and metabolic activity. Environmental temperature variations may be circadian, circannual, or geographic. Diurnal ranges of 35°C are commonly recorded in continental hot deserts. The largest circannual temperature variations occur in the centre of large land masses (for example, N.E. Asia) where winters fall to −65°C and summers have a mean of +20°C. Geographically, individual human populations live in environmental temperatures ranging from −65°C (January in Yakutsk) to +50°C (July in the Sahara). Metabolic heat production is similarly variable. Pressing a lift button may generate 1–2 kJ; walking up five flights of stairs may produce nearer 100 kJ.

Homeothermy is dependent upon continual thermoregulation. Specifically, a stable core temperature requires the balancing of heat gained by the body with heat lost to the environment. The individual components of the 'heat balance equation' are shown in Fig. 6.1. Most of the heat 'gained' by the body will normally come from metabolic heat production (see above). However, if ambient temperature exceeds skin temperature, the body will also gain heat from the environment. Hence, the need for '±' in Fig. 6.1. Heat losses occur by simple physical processes from skin to air (that is, conduction, convection, radiation, and evaporation).

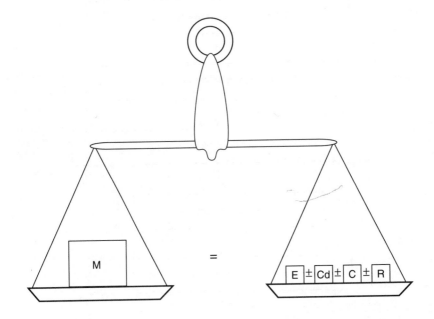

Fig. 6.1. The heat balance equation. M, metabolic heat production; E, evaporation (of sweat); Cd, conduction; C, convection; R, radiation.

6.1.1 Thermoregulation within the thermoneutral zone

There is a range of environmental temperatures over which it is relatively easy to maintain a stable core temperature. This is called the 'thermoneutral zone'. Here, metabolic heat production is minimal and thermoregulation is maintained by vasomotor activity (see below). In absolute terms the thermoneutral zone has been defined as 27–31°C for a naked 70 kg man. The lowest temperature within the thermoneutral zone is known as the 'critical temperature'. At ambient temperatures below this value, metabolic heat production has to be raised to offset heat losses. Clearly, with a critical temperature of 27°C, a naked person is poorly adapted to their environment, since few of the Earth's natural habitats provide an ambient temperature of this level throughout the day or year. In reality, of course, we make good use of clothing to provide insulation against heat loss from the body

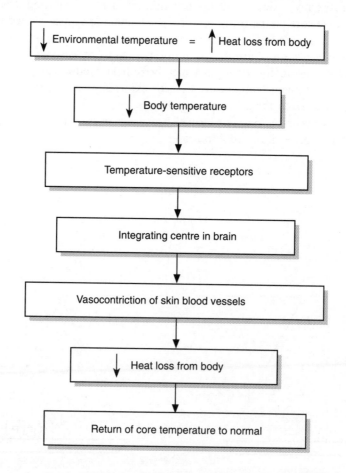

Fig. 6.2. Homeostatic control system reducing heat loss by peripheral vasoconstriction following a decreased environmental temperature.

(see p. 138). The critical temperature of a clothed individual would clearly be much lower than 27°C. However, since the precise value would vary considerably according to the amount and type of clothing worn, it still makes sense to define the thermoneutral zone in terms of a 'standard' naked individual.

Within the thermoneutral zone, minor changes in body temperature are compensated by simple constriction or dilatation of peripheral blood vessels. Peripheral vasoconstriction reduces the amount of blood moving from deep (warm) areas to the skin and, hence, less heat is lost to the environment. Peripheral vasodilatation has the opposite effect. Since blood flow in the skin can be regulated in the range 1–150 ml/min/100 g skin, such a mechanism is extremely effective. The responsiveness of the body's thermoregulatory system relies upon its ability to register temperature changes and subsequently correct any resultant deviation from the 'set point' (that is, normal body temperature). Figure 6.2 outlines the components of the feedback regulatory system whereby a reduction in environmental temperature results in peripheral vasoconstriction. It is a good example of a homeostatic control system, demonstrating two general principles of homeostasis. First, the 'regulated variable' exerts a key influence on its own control. Thus, a change in body temperature is the trigger for a sequence of events which ultimately restores body temperature to normal. Second, feedback is negative. Thus, a *decrease* in body temperature initiates a response that ultimately *increases* body temperature.

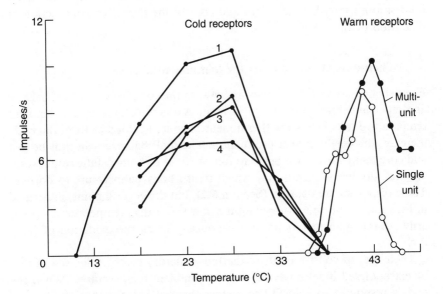

Fig. 6.3. Static discharge of cold and warm receptors as a function of skin temperature. From Iggo, A. (1969). *J. Physiology*, **200**, p. 418. Fig. 10—with permission.

The temperature-sensitive receptors shown in Fig. 6.2 are located both peripherally and centrally. Peripheral receptors are found in the skin and certain mucous membranes. Their density varies from approximately 18/cm² on the lips to one-tenth of this value on the palm of the hand. Peripheral receptors compromise two populations, one stimulated by a lower range of temperatures ('cold' receptors, Aδ fibres) and the other by a higher range of temperatures ('warm receptors', C fibres). Cold receptors outnumber warm receptors by approximately ten to one. Figure 6.3 shows how the static discharge of cold and warm receptors varies with skin temperature. The mid-point of the overlap of the two curves (33–35°C) represents the preferred mean skin temperature of a naked subject (see p. 153). Cold and warm receptors show different dynamic responses: the discharge from the former increases as skin temperature falls, whereas that from the latter increases as skin temperature rises.

Central receptors present in the hypothalamus and spinal cord measure core temperature. Like their peripheral counterparts, they comprise cold and warm receptors. The latter are thought to be located primarily in the hypothalamus. Information from peripheral and central thermoreceptors is transmitted to the hypothalamus and other integrating areas of the brain. In general, the pre-optic region and anterior hypothalamus mediate responses that result in heat loss, whereas cells within the posterior hypothalamus are involved in heat production and conservation. Efferent pathways run to the various effector organs described (Sections 6.2 and 6.3). Those regulating peripheral blood flow comprise sympathetic fibres which innervate arteriolar smooth muscle in the skin and control the degree of constriction or dilatation of the vessels.

6.1.2 Thermoregulation outside the thermoneutral zone

Figure 6.4 describes the relationship between the components of heat balance and environmental temperature in man. As mentioned above, if ambient temperature falls below the thermoneutral zone, heat losses from the body increase, outweighing heat production. Thermal 'balance' will thus be lost and core temperature will begin to fall. A series of homeostatic responses is very rapidly brought into play which return body temperature to normal. These responses are detailed (Section 6.2), but the general point, illustrated in Fig. 6.4, is that thermoregulation below the critical temperature is primarily reliant upon metabolic heat produced during the oxidation of body fuels.

There are, of course, limits to thermoregulatory control; Fig. 6.4 cannot be extrapolated indefinitely to very low ambient temperatures. When the body's responses to cold fail to restore thermal balance, deep body temperature falls. The clinical definition of hypothermia in man is a core temperature of 35°C or below.

At the upper end of the thermoneutral zone (above 31 °C in a naked 70 kg man), thermal 'balance' is again threatened. This time, heat gains (from the environment and metabolic processes) outweigh heat losses and core temperatures begin to rise. Once more a series of homeostatic responses is brought into play to return body temperature to normal. Figure 6.4 indicates the importance of evaporative heat loss mechanisms (mainly sweating in humans, see p. 147) in thermoregulation above the thermoneutral zone. Evaporation of water from the body surface results in loss of heat because of the large amount of energy (2510 kJ/l) needed to transform water into water vapour. Again, however, there are limits to thermoregulatory control and when the body's responses to heat fail to restore thermal balance, core

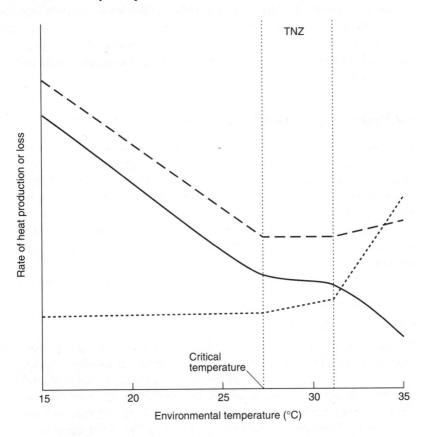

Fig. 6.4. The components of heat balance at different environmental temperatures. Metabolic heat production (– – –), non-evaporative heat loss (——), and evaporative heat loss (------). TNZ is the thermoneutral zone (the environmental temperature range over which metabolic rate is constant, and thermoregulation is by vasomotor activity). Critical temperature is the lowest temperature within the TNZ. Values apply to a naked 70 kg male. Factors such as clothing, posture, humidity, and air velocity will alter the absolute values shown.

temperature rises. The clinical definition of hyperthermia in humans is a deep body temperature of 40°C or above.

Physiological responses to cold and heat are, therefore, quite different, and will be described separately in this chapter. However, 'acclimatization' is relevant to both responses. Acclimatization is a term used to describe the physiological changes induced in a person following repeated exposure to altered environmental conditions. In the natural world it is rare to find a single environmental condition altering in isolation. Thus, changes in ambient temperature may often be accompanied by altered pressure or humidity. However, in the controlled environment of the laboratory it is relatively easy to alter experimentally a single environmental factor (for example, temperature). 'Acclimation' is the term used to describe physiological changes produced under these circumstances. Both 'acclimation' and 'acclimatization' should be distinguished from the term 'adaptation', which strictly describes an evolutionary change in the genome to an altered environmental variable.

6.2 Responses to low temperature

The homeostatic responses evoked by a low environmental temperature fall into two major categories. Some are designed to increase heat production, others to decrease heat loss. An alternative approach is to simply allow core temperature to drop. This response, however, although characteristic of hibernating mammals, is rare in humans. Cold responses are not exclusively physiological; many are behavioural. Indeed, moving into a warm room will often do more to maintain core temperature than any amount of vasoconstriction.

6.2.1 Increased heat production

6.2.1.1 *Increased activity*

The stamping of feet and rubbing of hands, much evident amongst football spectators at midwinter games, is a good example of increased activity in response to lowered ambient temperatures. Indeed, in most mammals, movement in general varies inversely with the temperature of the environment. In other words, we walk around quicker in winter than in summer! This increased voluntary muscle activity increases heat production by stimulating ATP hydrolysis on contraction of the muscle fibres (see Chapter 11).

Shivering is a specialized form of muscular activity which increases heat production in the same ways as exercise. It differs from the above examples, however, because it is predominantly an involuntary process. In humans, shivering is probably the most important physiological mechanism which initially offsets heat losses at low ambient temperatures. The term 'shivering' includes grades of muscular contraction which range from an increased muscle tone (pre-shivering tone), via a barely perceptible tremor, to vigorous overt shivering. Unlike normal muscle contraction, shivering consists of an uncoordinated pattern of activity in which muscle fibres contract and relax out of phase with one another. There is no purposeful movement.

Shivering is first apparent in the extensor muscles and proximal muscles of the upper limbs and trunk, rather than in the extremities. In advanced cases, the jaw muscles join in the act so that teeth start to chatter. (Interestingly, the word 'shiver' originates from the Middle English 'chivere' which, in turn, stems from the Old English for 'jaw'.) Shivering can increase heat production five-fold in humans, but it is both exhausting and a burden on energy reserves. It cannot, therefore, be sustained over long periods. Moreover, the tremor produced may increase convectional heat loss to the environment, which will reduce the efficiency of the process. This is particularly relevant in individuals with a large surface area to volume ratio (that is, small and immature forms such as children).

Both peripheral and central thermoreceptors influence the onset and extent of the shivering response. However, skin receptors appear to provide the main stimulus. If these stimuli are absent, shivering does not readily occur with a moderate fall in core temperature. Although the shivering response is well-developed in adults, it is often poorly developed or absent in neonates (see Chapter 2). Here, non-shivering thermogenesis may be of primary importance.

6.2.1.2 *Non-shivering thermogenesis*

Non-shivering thermogenesis is, as its name implies, a heat-producing mechanism which liberates energy through processes not involving muscular contraction. It is the process by which basal metabolic rate is largely maintained and can be increased in order to raise the metabolic rate two- to three-fold.

Brown adipose tissue has long been considered the major thermogenic tissue of the rat and, by implication, of other mammalian species as well. However, although there is little doubt that brown fat contributes to non-shivering thermogenesis in most newborn mammals (see Chapter 2), only in hibernators (see p. 140), bats, and rodents does the tissue persist throughout the life of the animal. This clearly sets a serious problem in evaluating the thermogenic role of brown fat in adult humans. In species which possess little functional brown adipose tissue as adults, other tissues such as skeletal muscle and liver are also involved in non-shivering thermogenesis. In absolute terms the thermogenic capacity of resting skeletal muscle is much lower than that for brown fat: assuming a standard mean energy value of 20 kJ/l oxygen at STP, the value for skeletal muscle is approximately 2 W/kg and that for brown fat nearer 300 W/kg. However, because of the larger mass of muscle, it can still make a significant thermogenic contribution. Indeed, in the rat, where brown fat persists into adulthood, the tissue forms less than 1 per cent of total body mass. In comparison, skeletal muscle represents over 40 per cent.

The biochemistry of brown fat thermogenesis and its stimulation by noradrenalin is discussed in Chapter 2. There are two explanations for thermogenesis by brown fat. One is that mitochondrial phosphorylation is uncoupled from respiration by the presence of large amounts of non-esterified fatty acids. The energy is thus lost directly as heat. The other explanation suggests an increased turnover of ATP via substrate recycling (originally called 'futile cycles'). In brown fat, recycling of triglycerides and fatty acids occurs; lipolysis and re-esterification processes result in ATP hydrolysis and heat production. This latter process is stimulated by noradrenalin. Skeletal muscle is also thought to use substrate cycles to generate heat. Catecholamines are again implicated in the response. Other hormones with a known calorigenic action include thyroid hormones, adrenocorticotrophic hormone (ACTH), glucagon, insulin, and corticosteroids. The major role of thyroid hormones lies in their control of endothermic thermogenesis (that is, metabolic reactions essential for the warm-blooded state). Thyroid hormones react with nuclear and mitochondrial T_3 receptors in most tissues (including muscle) to bring about changes in the properties and overall mass of mitochondria and in the activity of membrane-bound Na^+K^+-ATPase. The physiological role of this action is to set metabolic heat production at a level which balances heat loss within the thermoneutral zone. In experimental animals and human neonates, thyroid hormones also play a permissive role in cold-induced thermogenesis by increasing the responsiveness of tissues (primarily brown fat) to the thermogenic effect of catecholamines. This response, however, is of little significance in adult humans. The contribution of other 'calorigenic' hormones to normal thermoregulation is uncertain.

6.2.1.3 *Metabolic acclimatization and adaptation*

Most homeotherms show a significant increase in non-shivering thermogenesis in response to repeated exposure to low environmental temperatures. However, although many cold-chamber experiments have been carried out in humans, only a few have demonstrated changes which could be interpreted as true acclimatization. This may be due to the reluctance of 'volunteers' to endure sufficiently severe cold exposure for long periods of time. Indeed, where some degree of cold acclimatization has been demonstrated, the information has usually been obtained from polar explorers who have spent up to a year in the Arctic or Antarctic. Figure 6.5 presents the results of such a study. Members of an Australian Antarctic expedition were examined in a cold chamber in Melbourne before departure and then under similar conditions during their year in the Antarctic. In the Melbourne test, core temperature fell in the cold chamber. After 6 months in the Antarctic, this response was reversed. The implications are, therefore, for an increased metabolic response to cold due to enhanced non-shivering thermogenesis.

In animals which retain some brown fat into adulthood, cold acclimation results in a proliferation of the tissue and a general stimulation of sympathetic activity. For example, cold acclimation augments catecholamine-stimulated oxygen consumption of skeletal muscle in rats; it also increases the activity of the thyroid gland. There is no evidence for the regeneration of brown fat in adult humans during cold acclimatization. Neither is there good evidence that thyroid hormones play a major role in prolonged exposure to cold. The enhanced non-shivering thermogenesis seen in the polar explorers in Fig. 6.5 is likely to involve tissues such as skeletal muscle and liver. There is some evidence for an enhanced sensitivity to the calorigenic effect of noradrenalin in humans following cold acclimatization.

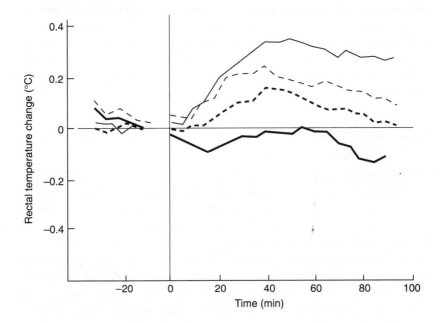

Fig. 6.5. Effect of acclimation to cold on core temperature. A group of Australians were placed in a cold room at time zero and exposed to standardized cold conditions: in Melbourne (——), after arrival in Antarctica (------), 6 months after arrival in Antarctica (——), and 12 months in Antarctica (------). Adapted from Budd, G.M. (1964). *Australian National Antarctic Research Expedition (ANARE) report series B*, **IV**, 35. Reproduced in Edholm, O.G. (1978). *Man—hot and cold*. Edward Arnold, London, with permission.

Eskimos and the Alakaluf Indians of Tierra del Fuego are two cold-dwelling populations who have been examined for possible metabolic adaptations to cold. The latter group traditionally sleep naked in simple shelters in ambient temperatures of 2–5°C. They do not shiver. Instead their survival appears to rely upon a basal metabolic rate some 30–40 per cent higher than in other populations. They have, therefore, developed a heritable adaptation to cold. Eskimos exhibit a similar adaptation, although it is not certain whether this is a true response to cold or the result of their traditionally high protein diet (see below) or both. There is no evidence of the persistence of brown fat in adult Eskimos.

6.2.1.4 *Increased feeding*

Appetite is stimulated by a cold environment and the increased food intake in turn elevates metabolic heat production. The increased metabolism is mainly caused by the protein content of the diet which results in an increased substrate recycling of amino acids. Thus, the traditional high-protein diet of Eskimos contributes to their elevated basal metabolism and helps offset heat losses in the cold. However, increased metabolism after feeding is also accompanied by an increased blood flow to the peripheral regions of the body. This inevitably increases heat losses to the environment (see p. 150) and, consequently, reduces the thermoregulatory contribution of feeding.

6.2.2 **Decreased heat loss**

6.2.2.1 *Behaviour*

The importance of behaviour in thermoregulation is often overlooked and the behavioural responses to cold, particularly in extreme conditions, are at least as important as the physiological responses discussed above. Indeed, many adult mammals, although fully capable of shivering and vasoconstricting, preferentially use behavioural means of elevating body temperature when experimentally stressed. Humans are no exception: our primary behavioural response to cold is one of avoidance. In extreme climates our schedule of daily activities often reflects our dislike of low temperatures. For example, inhabitants of the Andes in South America rise at dawn and go to bed at sunset: most of the working day is spent out of doors taking advantage of the solar radiation. Andean children are placed in the sun during the day and in communal beds at night. Heat losses in a cold environment may also be offset by reducing the surface area available for heat exchange. Thus, we, like other mammals, 'huddle' in low temperatures, curling up like a ball with arms folded across the body and legs bent up. Rat pups, with little autonomic capacity for thermoregulation have been shown to regulate body temperature by controlling the compactness of the huddle.

6.2.2.2 *Insulation* – Esky Mo fur in coat.

Most terrestrial mammals use fur for insulation. Fur insulates by trapping air next to the skin, thereby reducing convectional heat losses to the environment. The insulative value of fur is directly related to its length. Cold-adapted species therefore have thicker coats. They also tend to have larger frames to support the fur. A mouse with a 15 cm fur coat would clearly have mobility problems! The insulation provided by fur is usually varied to match seasonal temperature changes. Thus, many mammals moult in spring. Sudden decreases in ambient temperature are combated by erection of the fur (horripilation) which increases the amount of air trapped by the hairs. 'Goose pimples' are the most noticeable result of horripilation in humans; low environmental temperatures cause the contraction of the pilo-erector muscles of the few hairs that are present.

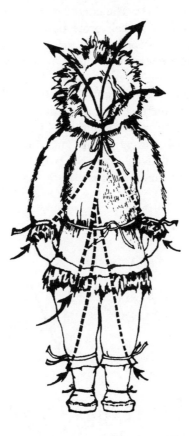

Fig. 6.6. The traditional Eskimo clothing is multilayered with a windproof outer layer. Vents in the clothing can be opened or closed with drawstrings to vary insulation with activity. Reprinted from Moran, E.F. (1979). *Human adaptability: an introduction to ecological anthropology.* By permission of Westview Press, Boulder, Colorado.

In the absence of fur, clothing provides us with our main protection against cold. There are several parallels to be drawn between the roles of clothing and fur. Thus, the insulation of clothing is again provided by trapped air, this time between the fibres of the clothing fabric. As with fur, the thermal insulation of clothing is proportional to the thickness of the trapped air. This is enhanced if several layers of clothing are worn with a windproof outer garment. The latter must not be completely impermeable to water vapour, however or the insulation value of the clothing would be decreased by condensation (see p. 144) and possible freezing of evaporated sweat. As with fur, the insulation provided by clothing must be variable in order to match changing activity and heat production. This is facilitated by the use of multilayered garments. In addition, traditional Eskimo clothing has many vented openings which can be released or closed with drawstrings to lose or conserve body heat (Fig. 6.6). The extremities of the body present special problems (see p. 143). The hands, feet, and head, thus, require the most specialized clothing for their protection.

Subcutaneous fat also affords some protection against the cold and in temperate races there are seasonal changes in body weight, with an increase in the winter and decrease in summer (Fig. 6.7). However, these changes (1–2 kg) are too small to significantly affect overall thermal balance and may simply reflect an increased food consumption (see p. 136), reduced activity, or both, during winter months. There is also little evidence for extra insulation in cold-stressed populations. Indeed, Eskimos, Alacalufs, and Andeans are all relatively lean. Nevertheless, in general terms these races do have a shorter, more compact body shape (and, hence, a smaller

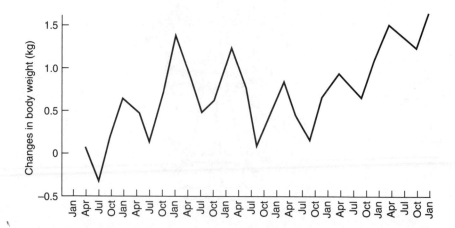

Fig. 6.7. Seasonal changes in body weight of human subjects from surveys conducted over 7 years. Note that body weight peaks in winter months. Adapted from Harries, J.M. and Hollingsworth, D.F. (1953). *British Medical Journal*, **1**, 75–8, with permission.

surface area) when compared to their tropical counterparts (contrast an Eskimo with a member of a West African tribe). Eskimos are traditionally described as showing other 'morphological adaptations' to cold, including eyefold characteristics and facial flatness, but it is unlikely that these will afford any significant protection against cold stress.

The foregoing account of the relative insulative properties of fur and clothing is relevant only to terrestrial life. In water the insulation values of clothing and fur decline, because the insulator itself (air) is lost or at best compressed. The section on hypothermia in cold water (p. 143) discusses the special problems of immersion in cold water. Finally, it is pertinent to stress the importance of housing and shelter. Like clothing, housing must retain heat and be windproof. In a cold climate protection against wind has very high priority both in the design of houses and clothing. The concept of the 'wind chill factor' in relation to thermal comfort is discussed in the section on thermal comfort (p. 154).

6.2.2.3 *Cutaneous vasoconstriction*

The primary physiological response to a reduced environmental temperature involves a cutaneous vasoconstriction. As detailed on p. 129, a decreased blood flow through the cutaneous circulation reduces convectional heat

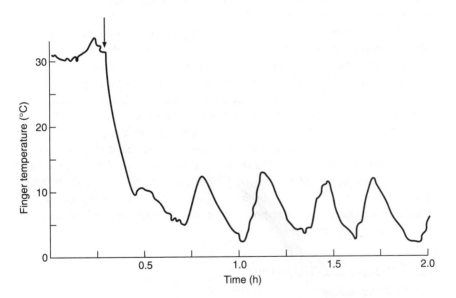

Fig. 6.8. Record of a hunting reaction in a human subject. The subject's hand was immersed in ice at −5°C at time zero (arrowed) and finger temperature was recorded over the following 90 min. Room temperature was 15°C. From Werner, J. (1977). *Pflügers Archives*, **367**, 291–4. Reproduced by permission of Springer-Verlag, Heidelberg.

losses from the surface of the skin. Vasoconstriction results from an increased sympathetic activity to the blood vessels in the skin. Although the initial response to cold is that of a cutaneous vasoconstriction, prolonged cooling results in a paradoxical vasodilatation with a consequent heat loss. Thereafter, vasoconstriction alternates with periods of vasodilatation (see Fig. 6.8.). This so-called 'hunting reaction' is found primarily in the extremities of the body where there is little metabolically active tissue. The phenomenon serves to prevent tissue damage (for example, frostbite) by severe cold (see p. 143). Cold vasodilatation represents a general dilatation of all skin blood vessels, including an opening of the arteriovenous anastamoses. It results primarily from a direct cold-induced paralysis of the peripheral blood vessels which lose their ability to respond to noradrenalin at low temperatures.

6.2.2.4 *Vascular acclimatization and adaptation*

Although evidence for physiological acclimatization to heat is readily obtainable (see p. 149) similar evidence with respect to cold is harder to come by. There is some indication for local acclimatization to cold in the fingers and hands of people regularly exposed to low temperatures (fishermen, polar explorers, etc.). Here the initial vasoconstrictor response to cold (see above) is less severe and the onset of the subsequent vasodilatation more rapid than in unacclimatized subjects.

Eskimos also exhibit a higher than normal rate of peripheral blood flow to their extremities when exposed to cold. Moreover, they show an altered cardiovascular response to face cooling. Immersion of the face in cold water normally causes a reflex bradycardia and vasoconstriction of the hands. In Eskimo subjects this response is greatly reduced or absent. Clearly these examples represent true low temperature adaptations which will both prevent injury and permit greater manual dexterity in a cold environment. A different type of vascular adaptation is seen in the diving women of Korea and Japan (Ama). These women dive for shellfish and edible seaweeds in water temperatures of 10°C, wearing only minimal clothing. Skin temperatures appear to be maintained without increasing peripheral blood flow. Instead a greater proportion of the venous return is channelled through subcutaneous vessels.

6.2.3. **Reduced body temperature**

6.2.3.1 *Hibernation*

Maintenance of a core temperature of 36–38°C in conditions of extreme cold is expensive metabolically. In small mammals with high metabolic rates, a further increase may be impossible when food is scarce or unobtainable. Under such circumstances, some mammals opt out of homeothermy and allow their core temperature to fall to a level approaching that of the environment. This eliminates the increased cost of keeping warm and, since cold tissues use less fuel, energy reserves last longer. As body temperature falls, heart rate, metabolic rate, and other physiological variables will be correspondingly reduced. Despite this, the animal retains the ability to rewarm itself to its original temperature without relying on heat from the environment.

This phenomenon of hibernation is not simply a failure to thermoregulate in the cold. Rather, it is a precisely regulated physiological process. Entry into hibernation is a long process which can last several days or weeks. It is governed by several environmental factors including ambient temperature, availability of food and water, and time of year (light:dark period is especially relevant). It is also thought to have an endogenous (hormonal) component. Arousal from the hibernation is relatively quick; core temperature may be raised by 30°C in as little as 90 min. Arousal is primarily dependent upon ambient temperature. It is, however, expensive metabolically, employing both shivering and non-shivering thermogenesis (see p. 133). The latter involves brown adipose tissue, which is retained in the adult hibernator.

6.2.3.2 *Reduced body temperature in humans*

A reduced body temperature in response to cold is comparatively rare in humans. Nevertheless, two natural populations (Australian Aborigines and the Bushmen of the Kalahari desert in Africa) demonstrate the beginnings of a hypothermic response to a lowered environmental temperature. Figure 6.9 contrasts the responses of male Aborigines and (white) Europeans to a night of moderate cold exposure. During the night, the core temperature of the Europeans initially fell but was maintained just above 36°C by shivering and an increased metabolism. In contrast, the Aborigines allowed their deep body temperature to fall below 35°C without attempting to compensate for heat losses. A similar response is seen amongst Kalahari Bushmen. One can speculate teleologically about these responses. Thus, the Aborigine and Kalahari Bushman can afford to cool down during the night as they will quickly warm up again in the morning sun. This could never be guaranteed in Europe! The nocturnal hypothermic response may therefore be seen as an adaptation to reduce the metabolic costs of keeping warm in natural populations who normally experience cold nights and warm days.

6.2.4 **Failure to thermoregulate in extreme cold**

Up to now we have considered how the body manages to maintain thermal balance in the face of a reduced ambient temperature. However, under conditions of extreme cold, the normal thermoregulatory mechanisms may fail and give rise to special problems of cold stress. Hypothermia and cold injury are two such problems.

6.2.4.1 *Hypothermia*

It is surprisingly difficult to reduce core temperature below 35.5°C because of the effectiveness of the behavioural responses and shivering mechanism described earlier. However, if core temperature does drop below 35°C, the ensuing muscular weakness will result in a decreased mobility and diminished shivering. In the absence of these heat generating processes, core temperatures will rapidly fall further. At temperatures below 34°C mental

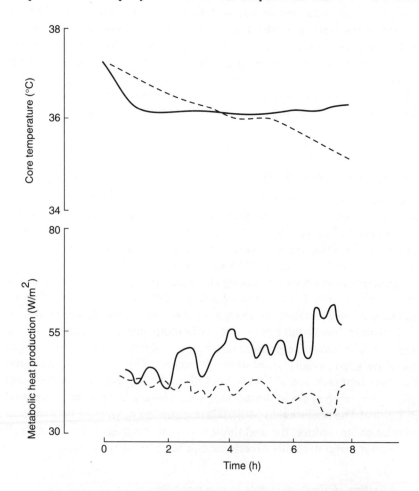

Fig. 6.9. Reduced body temperature in man. Response of a group of male Aborigines (------) and Europeans (——) to a night of moderate cold exposure. From Richards, S.A. (1973). *Temperature regulation.* Wykeham Publications, Taylor & Francis, London.

confusion and visual disturbances occur. Consciousness may be lost between 32 and 30°C. In hypothermia the most important effects of a reduced body temperature are on the heart. At core temperatures below 28°C cardiac arrhythmias occur and ventricular fibrillation is often responsible for fatalities at these temperatures. Cold also slows the pacemaker and cardiac output declines, primarily due to a reduced heart rate. Under such circumstances it may not be possible to maintain adequate blood flow to the coronary and/or cerebral circulations.

Recovery from severe hypothermia can be rapid and complete. The lowest core temperature from which anyone has survived is 18°C observed in a woman who was buried in a snowdrift for several hours. However, there is considerable individual variation in the ability both to develop and survive hypothermia. A high level of physical fitness is important since a high rate of energy expenditure (necessary to offset heat losses) can be maintained for longer without fatigue. Survival is further complicated if clothing becomes soaked with rain or sweat. Under these circumstances the insulation is much reduced since the thermal conductivity of water is far greater than that of air. Similar problems accelerate hypothermia following immersion in cold water (see p. 144). Finally, those at the extremes of age are at greater risk from accidental hypothermia. In the neonate, for example, temperature-regulating mechanisms are not fully developed; in the elderly, hypothalamic control is impaired. The special problems of thermoregulation in the young and old are discussed in detail in Chapters 2 and 5.

6.2.4.2 *Cold injury*

Frostbite is the most serious form of cold injury, characterized by a freezing of peripheral tissues. In mild cases of frostbite, only the skin freezes. On thawing the injured tissue simply peels off and is replaced by new growth. However, in more severe cases, deeper tissues, including muscle, bone, and tendon may also freeze. Damage to the affected cells results from the mechanical action of ice crystals and also from cell dehydration. Ice forming within cells reduces cellular water content and, therefore, increases osmolality. In addition to general cellular damage, the permeability of blood vessels is increased by freezing. On thawing there is a consequent loss of fluid from the circulation into tissue spaces. The increase in packed cell volume within the vessels of the affected tissue then reduces or even stops blood flow and gangrene may result, with the loss of fingers, toes, or even hands and feet. The best treatment for frostbite is to warm the affected part gradually so that damaged capillaries do not rupture when blood returns.

A prolonged cooling (as opposed to freezing) of the feet and legs in cold water can result in peripheral vasoneuropathy. The problem arises as a consequence of a reduced blood flow due to prolonged cold vasoconstriction. Although gangrene may ensue, the main damage is neuromuscular.

Sensory and motor paralysis in the early stages of immersion injury are due to the direct effects of cold on nerve and muscle. Finally, chilblains are a mild form of cold injury, occurring in fingers, toes, or ears. They occur following prolonged cooling of the extremities, particularly in individuals with a poor circulation. Affected parts become hyperaemic, tender, and itchy.

6.2.5 Hypothermia in cold water

Major heat losses in water are by conduction. Moreover, the higher thermal conductivity of water compared to air means that the rate of heat loss is greatly increased in an aquatic environment. Indeed, accidental deaths in water are thought to result as much from immersion hypothermia as from drowning. The hypothermic effects of cold water have been studied in some detail. Survival time varies directly with water temperature. For example, a naked person will become hypothermic after 20–30 min in water at 5°C and after 1.5–2 hours in water at 15°C. These temperatures approximate the mean sea temperatures around the coast of Britain during January and July respectively.

Increased insulation prolongs survival time. As mentioned above (see p. 139) normal clothes are rather ineffective insulators in water. However, subcutaneous fat provides some insulation. Many aquatic mammals (for example, seals and whales) use blubber effectively to reduce heat losses in

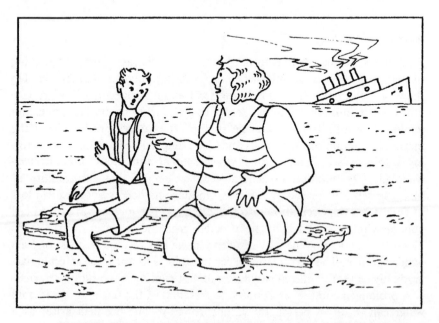

Fig. 6.10. 'You stay here, George—I'll be back with help in no time!' (With apologies to Donald McGill.)

cold seas. Any increased weight afforded by the fat is supported by the water. Terrestrial mammals, including humans, have smaller subcutaneous fat deposits to facilitate mobility. Nevertheless, fat does afford some protection against heat losses in water, so that, in general, thin people become hypothermic in water more rapidly than fat people. Indeed, a study of cross-channel swimmers who survived for up to 20 h in sea temperatures of 15–17°C showed that all of those who were successful were fat.

Heat losses in water are affected by the degree of movement of the subject. By remaining still, the water in immediate contact with the body surface becomes warmed just as the layer of air round the body is heated by convective heat losses on land. Weak swimming or struggling disturbs the warmed layers and therefore increases heat losses still further. Hence, those in potential danger of shipwreck in cold waters are advised to float with a life jacket or wreckage and await rescue rather than attempt to swim any great distance to shore. The exception may be the obese individual who also happens to be a strong swimmer (Fig. 6.10).

6.3 Responses to high temperature

If human life evolved in Central Africa, as many evolutionists argue, this may well explain why we appear so well adapted to life in a hot climate. Central to this adaptation is a very efficient sweating mechanism (see p. 147) which maintains thermal balance by increasing heat loss. However, few natural populations live in conditions where the ambient temperature exceeds core temperature by more than 12°C. This contrasts strongly with our ability to survive at temperatures up to 80°C below deep body temperature. Overheating appears to be more of a problem than overcooling. Indeed, death may ensue with a rise in core temperature of only 5°C as against a fall of more than twice this value.

Responses to high temperatures fall into two major categories. Some are designed to decrease heat gain (both from endogenous production and external sources), others to increase heat loss. Heat responses are often the converse of what happens in the cold (for example, vasodilatation vs vasoconstriction). As with cold responses, altered behaviour is often as important as altered physiology when ambient temperatures start to rise.

6.3.1 Decreased heat gain

6.3.1.1 *Reduced activity*

An increased voluntary muscle activity increases heat production (see p. 132). Not surprisingly, therefore, general apathy and inertia are synonymous with hot climates. Manual work is normally confined to the cooler parts of the day. Some mammals reduce their activity to zero in the summer months and remain dormant in their burrows, thereby reducing the costs of staying cool. This type of dormancy is known as 'aestivation' (from the Latin 'aestas', meaning 'summer') in contrast to 'hibernation' (see p. 140).

6.3.1.2 *Reduced feeding*

An increased food intake elevates metabolic heat production (see p. 136). Not surprisingly, a hot environment promotes anorexia. Food preference is often directed towards items with a high water content (for example, fruit and salad vegetables) as stimulation of the thirst mechanism attempts to offset potential dehydration in the heat.

6.3.1.3 *Reduced heat gain from the environment*

The importance of behaviour in reducing heat gains from the environment is evident from a study of lifestyle in the tropics. Thus, manual workers start work much earlier in the day than they do in more temperate regions and break off work when it starts to get hot. Extended lunch breaks and siestas are part of the culture in hot climates. Clothing and housing provide the major insulation against solar radiation, just as they protect us from cold (see p. 138). However, it is difficult to keep external heat out without also preventing loss of internal (metabolic) heat. This may, in part, explain why overheating is a more critical problem than overcooling. The use of clothing varies between areas of dry and humid heat. In dry desert areas, clothing serves both to reduce heat gain from the environment and increase heat loss from the body. This is achieved by the use of loose fitting, lightweight, light coloured materials. These reflect much of the short-wave solar radiation, but also permit the circulation of air necessary to evaporate sweat. Clothing is also important in coping with hot desert winds. This is one of the most serious problems faced by desert populations, since it will lower the threshold to dry heat by accelerating the dehydration process (see also p. 151). Humid, tropical regions present different problems. Here sweating is much less efficient in removing heat from the body because evaporation is retarded. Under these circumstances minimal clothing is worn to reduce the body's heat load and maximize the surface area for sweat evaporation.

Housing in hot (dry) areas is constructed with the same objectives in mind as desert clothing. Heat gain from the environment is minimized by the use of compact designs which reduce the surface area exposed to the heat. Subterranean dwellings are constructed in extreme deserts to take advantage of the heat capacity of the earth itself. Rooms in Matmata houses in the Saraha, for example, are built 10 m underground. They remain remarkably cool. One real problem in hot dry areas is the large diurnal temperature variation resulting from the lack of atmospheric moisture and cloud cover. Diurnal ranges of 35°C are commonly recorded in continental hot deserts.

Azizia in Tripoli, North Africa, once recorded 52°C and −3°C during the same 24 h, a record diurnal range. In such conditions, building materials with a high heat capacity (for example, adobe, mud, and stone) are useful because they can absorb heat in the day and radiate it at night.

6.3.2 Increased heat loss

6.3.2.1 *Body shape*

The 'ideal' body shape for hot desert conditions is tall with long lean limbs and low subcutaneous fat. Tallness maximizes the surface area to body weight ratio for evaporative cooling, while leanness facilitates heat conduction from deep body tissues. The Nilotic people of the Sudan and the Masai of Kenya whose adult males average 2.14 m in height are often cited as examples of the optimal human form for the desert environment.

6.3.2.2 *Sweating*

Sweating is the primary means of increasing heat loss as environmental temperature rises. The human body has approximately 2 million sweat glands. Although this averages 120 sweat glands per cm^2, in fact, the sweat glands are not evenly distributed throughout the body and 50 per cent of the total sweat production comes from the chest and back. Humans can produce more sweat per unit area of skin than any other mammal (even pigs!). The maximum sweat rate in man is around 3 l/h. However, this cannot be sustained for long periods of time, so that a typical value for a man working in hot dry conditions would be nearer 12 l/day.

Women, in general, have lower sweat rates than men. The contention that 'a man sweats, but a lady perspires' has some physiological basis, since a man produces up to twice as much sweat as a woman when exposed to a comparable heat load. Controlled hyperthermic experiments have also revealed striking differences in the absolute sweat rate between indigenous populations of hot countries. Native tribes of New Guinea, for example, have much lower sweat rates than either Nigerians or Europeans when studied under similar conditions.

Sweat itself is a hypotonic solution produced by eccrine glands in the dermis of the skin. A primary isotonic secretion produced by the proximal (coiled) region of the gland is subsequently modified by solute reabsorption as the fluid moves along the duct towards the skin surface. At low rates of secretion the sodium content of sweat is low (5 mmol/l) whereas at high secretion rates there is less time for ductal reabsorption and the sodium content can approach 10 times this value.

In order for heat to be lost, sweat must not only be secreted: it must evaporate. The latent heat of evaporation of water at 37°C is 2.4 kJ/ml. If evaporation occurs on the skin, the majority of this heat will come from the body itself. For a maximum sweat rate of 3 l/h, heat loss will, therefore, approximate 7000 kJ/h or 20 times the basal metabolic rate. The lack of hair on the surface of the human body clearly facilitates the evaporation of sweat, but the process is critically influenced by the amount of water vapour in the atmosphere. The human body appears dry in the desert because evaporation is so rapid that sweat vaporizes as soon as it reaches the surface of the skin. In tropical regions, however, where humidity approaches 100 per cent, little or no evaporation occurs, and so this method of losing heat is not available. Atmospheric humidity is clearly an essential consideration in any discussion of the role of sweating.

A critical factor in the use of sweating to combat a high heat load is the availability of water. As shown in Fig. 6.11, water requirements in hot climates vary according to the ambient temperature and level of activity. Where drinking water is unrestricted, a balance is soon established between fluid intake and the combined fluid losses of sweating and urinary excretion. Where water is restricted, varying degrees of dehydration occur. Normally, in humans, thirst mechanisms are triggered by a fluid loss of 2 per cent of

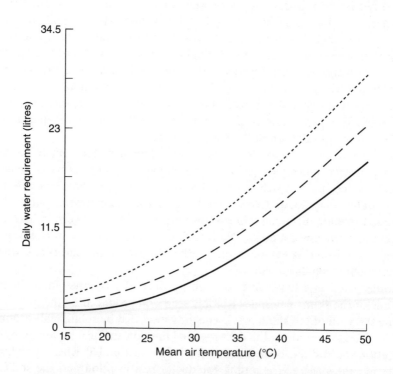

Fig. 6.11. Daily water requirements at different ambient temperatures for three levels of activity: at rest in the shade (——), undertaking moderate work in the sun (------), and undertaking hard work in the sun (······). From Lee, D.H.K. (1968). Man in the desert. In *Desert biology* (ed. G.W. Brown). Academic Press, NY, with permission.

the body weight. Urinary water losses are also reduced by increased secretion of antidiuretic hormone. The section on heat collapse (p. 152) considers in more detail the specific problems of water deficiency in hot climates.

Finally, since sodium chloride is a major constituent of sweat, excessive sweating may lead to a negative salt balance unless salt intake is increased. Visitors to hot climates are, therefore, often advised to supplement their diet with salt tablets. The body also counteracts salt losses by increasing its secretion of aldosterone which acts on the renal distal tubules, salivary, and sweat gland ducts to conserve sodium. The section on heat exhaustion (p. 151) considers in more detail the specific problems of salt deficiency in hot climates.

6.3.2.3 *Sweating and acclimatization*

Evidence for true physiological acclimatization to heat is much more readily obtainable than similar responses to cold (see p. 140). Indeed, all human populations will acclimatize to desert conditions within 1–2 weeks. Central to this acclimatization is an increased sweat rate. After 2 weeks in a hot climate, for example, sweat losses per unit time may have doubled compared to the initial exposure. Sweating also starts at a lower threshold core temperature and acclimatized individuals show a decreased salt concentration in sweat. This prevents some of the symptoms of salt-deficiency heat exhaustion (for example, muscular cramps; see p. 151). Acclimatization to heat varies with atmospheric humidity: the increase in sweating is much more marked in hot humid conditions than in hot dry climates.

6.3.2.4 *Panting and salivation*

Evaporative heat losses in humans are almost exclusively the result of sweating. Other mammals, with their fewer sweat glands and fur coats which impede evaporation, cool primarily by panting. This serves to increase evaporation from the upper respiratory tract. A heat-stressed dog increases its respiratory frequency 10-fold; humans examined under similar conditions show only a modest increase in ventilation.

There are several advantages of panting over sweating as a means of losing heat. First, the panting animal provides its own air currents to facilitate evaporation. Sweating, of course, is always reliant on external air movements which cannot be controlled. Secondly, panting does not result in the loss of sodium which inevitably accompanies sweating. Thirdly, venous drainage from the nasal passages of some panting animals serves to pre-cool arterial blood flowing to the brain and thereby prevent overheating of the brain. The major disadvantage of panting results from the increased ventilation which increases the work of breathing and causes alkalosis.

Finally, a few mammals spread saliva over their fur as an additional evaporative heat loss mechanism. This approach, however, although analogous to sweating in humans, is neither widespread nor very effective.

6.3.2.5 *Cardiovascular responses*

A rapid cutaneous vasodilatation occurs as ambient temperature rises. This promotes the transfer of heat from deep to superficial body tissues and, thence, to the environment. The homeostatic control system which reduces heat gain by peripheral vasodilatation is essentially the opposite of that shown in Fig. 6.2. If thermal balance is lost in the heat, core temperature starts to rise. Other cardiovascular changes then become apparent. Cardiac output, for example, increases. This is due initially to an increased heart rate, with temperature having a direct effect on the sinoatrial node. If heat stress is prolonged, however, an increased stroke volume may also occur. Changes in cardiac output have minimal effects on blood pressure because of the fall in peripheral resistance produced by the vasodilatation described above. During acclimatization to heat, some of the cardiovascular changes are reversed. Heart rate, for example, will fall if core temperature is normalized by increased sweating. Cardiac output will then return towards normal.

6.3.3 Hyperthermia and heat storage

Unlike humans, some mammals can withstand varying degrees of hyperthermia. The camel, for example, makes no attempt to thermoregulate until its core temperature exceeds 41°C, while fast-running African gazelles can tolerate a core temperature of 46°C for several hours. The brain temperature of these animals, however, is kept at 40°C by a special heat-exchange network at the base of the brain. This hyperthermic response to heat is analogous to the hypothermic response seen in cold-stressed hibernators (see p. 140) in as much as it reduces the costs of staying cool. In particular, much of the fluid normally lost in sweat will be conserved. For a camel weighing 500 kg, the amount of heat stored due to a 4°C temperature rise corresponds to over 7000 kJ. This is equivalent to a saving of 3 l of sweat, which will be particularly important if water supplies are restricted. At night, the stored heat can be unloaded by conduction and radiation with minimal fluid losses.

6.3.4 Failure to thermoregulate in extreme heat

Up to now we have considered how the body manages to maintain thermal balance in the face of increased environmental temperatures. However, under conditions of extreme heat, the normal thermoregulatory mechanisms may fail and give rise to special problems of heat stress. Heat stroke, heat exhaustion, and heat collapse are three conditions that fall into this category. Although such problems are normally associated with hot climates, they may also represent occupational problems (for example, for iron foundry workers) in more temperate areas of the world.

6.3.4.1 *Heat stroke*

Heat stroke is the most serious consequence of heat stress, resulting from a complete loss of thermoregulatory control. Although normally associated with life in the desert, heat stroke is occasionally a problem in more temperate regions. Initial characteristics of heat stroke are a loss of energy and irritability, but then follow serious neurological and mental disturbances. Sweating diminishes or ceases and the subject passes into a coma as core temperature rises to 42°C or beyond. Unless treatment is started immediately to lower body temperature, death usually ensues. The loss of thermoregulatory control in heat stroke appears to be due primarily to a failure of the sweating mechanism. This may be a complete failure due to hypothalamic malfunction or simply an inadequacy to meet the needs of the particular heat load. Cellular damage and coagulation of proteins both accompany very high core temperatures: post-mortem examination of heat stroke victims have revealed pathological changes in the CNS including neuronal degeneration.

6.3.4.2 *Heat exhaustion*

The symptoms of heat exhaustion vary according to the cause of the condition. Water-deficiency heat exhaustion, for example, results from insufficient water replacement of fluid losses. Most people can tolerate a 3–4 per cent water deficit. With a loss of 5–8 per cent, however, fatigue and dizziness set in; a loss of over 10 per cent causes physical and mental deterioration. The lethal limit for human dehydration is a fluid loss of 15–25 per cent of the body weight, a figure similar to that seen for a number of other mammals. Water deficiency initially affects the extracellular fluid volume but, if continued, intracellular dehydration ensues. A gradual decrease in plasma volume accompanies the dehydration and this is responsible for the initial symptoms. Later, cellular damage accompanies the increase in plasma osmolality.

Salt-deficiency heat exhaustion occurs when salt losses in sweat are not adequately replaced by salt in the diet. Tissue osmolality falls and extracellular compartments contract. The syndrome is characterized by heat cramps, usually in the legs, arms, or back and by fatigue and dizziness.

6.3.4.3 *Heat collapse*

Heat collapse or syncope is characterized by fatigue, dizziness, and a temporary loss of consciousness in the heat. The condition is caused by a pooling of blood in dilated blood vessels of skeletal muscles and skin in the lower limbs. The cerebral circulation is, therefore, compromised and consciousness slowly fades away. Heat collapse is a characteristic of the unacclimatized individual in a hot climate. It is also an occupational hazard of soldiers on sentry duty in more temperate climates during summer months. The problem, however, is usually self-correcting, since the fainting soldier has no choice but to fall down. Once horizontal, venous return will increase and the cerebral circulation will be re-established.

6.4 Thermal comfort

It is appropriate to conclude a chapter on thermoregulation with a short account of thermal comfort, since the attainment of comfort is the ultimate goal of all thermoregulatory processes. Thermal comfort is something everyone appreciates and understands but which is difficult to define satisfactorily. In practice the seven-point Bedford scale is often used, ranging from 'much too cool', through 'comfortable, neither cool nor warm' to 'much too warm'. In other words comfort is generally defined as a lack of discomfort! Relating such subjective feelings to physiological changes is not simple. Certainly we feel uncomfortable if we sweat profusely or shiver markedly, but discomfort is frequently experienced under less extreme conditions. Such discomfort depends upon the individual, the time of day or year, phase of the menstrual cycle, and the individual's recent thermal environment.

Thermal comfort can generally be related to skin temperature, particularly that of the face. Cold or hot skin is perceived as being uncomfortable when compared with skin of intermediate temperature. Skin temperature is determined by several factors, including radiant heat gain from or loss to the environment, ambient temperature, the rate of sweating (and, hence, ambient humidity), and air flow. These help to explain some cases of discomfort. For example, one is more likely to feel cold as the airflow increases and more likely to feel warm if the humidity is high with reduced evaporative heat loss.

However, there is also a relationship between skin and core temperature in any assessment of comfort. If the core temperature is above the thermoregulatory set point then a cooler environment is preferred for comfort. In contrast, if the core temperature is below the set point then a warmer environment is more comfortable. As a result, the same flow of air (with regard to speed, temperature, and humidity) is a 'balmy breeze' for a sunbather (picking up radiant heat) yet a 'draught' for somebody sitting in a room. This relationship also explains why, as the amount of physical work increases, the preferred ambient temperature decreases and the preferred air velocity increases. We can also understand why it is comforting to warm our hands in front of the fire on a winter evening or to have a nip of brandy (which warms the skin by cutaneous vasodilatation) before going out into the cold. In the latter case, however, the increased heat loss that this produces could be dangerous. In spite of these results, a person makes the *same* assessment of skin temperature whether he or she is hypothermic, euthermic, or hyperthermic. This is interpreted to indicate that changes in core temperature do not influence cutaneous sensitivity and input to the CNS, but rather the way it is interpreted.

In practice, cutaneous temperature is modified greatly by clothing (see p. 138) and it is the aim of this form of insulation to produce a comfortable microclimate in spite of an inclement environment. The preferred mean skin temperature in a nude subject is approximately 33°C—considerably higher

Estimated windspeed (mph) ⇩	Actual Thermometer reading (°C)											
	10	5	−1	−7	−12	−18	−24	−29	−35	−40	−46	−51
	Equivalent temperature (°C)											
Calm	10	5	−1	−7	−12	−18	−24	−29	−35	−40	−46	−51
5	9	3	−3	−9	−15	−21	−26	−32	−38	−44	−50	−56
10	5	−2	−9	−16	−23	−31	−36	−44	−50	−57	−64	−71
15	2	−6	−13	−21	−28	−36	−43	−50	−58	−66	−73	−81
20	0	−8	−16	−24	−32	−40	−48	−55	−64	−72	−80	−87
25	−1	−9	−18	−26	−34	−43	−51	−59	−67	−76	−84	−92
30	−2	−11	−19	−28	−36	−45	−53	−62	−71	−79	−88	−96
35	−3	−12	−20	−29	−38	−47	−55	−64	−73	−81	−90	−99
40	−4	−13	−21	−30	−39	−48	−57	−66	−74	−83	−92	−101

Windspeeds greater than 40 mph have little added effect — Little danger for properly clothed person, maximum danger of false sense of security — Increasing danger from freezing of exposed flesh — Great danger

Fig. 6.12. The wind chill effect. The cooling power of wind on exposed flesh expressed as equivalent temperature under calm conditions. To use the table, find the windspeed in the left-hand column and the actual temperature across the top. The intersection of the two columns gives the effective temperature acting on exposed skin. From *TB Med 81 (NAVMED P5052 29)* (1970). Department of Navy, Washington, DC.

than an ambient temperature of approximately 20°C that is acceptable to most sedentary persons dressed conventionally. Finally, attempts have been made to assess the 'comfort index' of an environment and to measure it objectively. This has led to the concept of the 'wind chill factor'. This is a measure of how much colder the air appears to be if it is moving—or a person is moving through it—compared to when it is still. Figure 6.12 details the cooling power of wind on exposed flesh expressed as an equivalent temperature under calm conditions. As a further refinement, tables have also been produced that include the effects of humidity and radiant heat, for example. In all cases, the amount of protection that is required for comfort can be estimated. Objective measurements of cooling effects due to air flow and evaporation and heat gains or losses by radiation, can all be measured by thermometers suitably modified for measuring each of these factors. However, the ultimate test must be the individual—only he or she can decide whether the circumstances are comfortable or not.

Further reading

Colquhoun, E.Q. and Clark, M.G. (1991). Has thermogenesis in muscle been overlooked and misinterpreted? *News in Physiological Sciences*, **6**, 256–9.

Edholm, O.G. (1978). *Man—hot and cold*. Institute of Biology, Studies in Biology, No. 97. Edward Arnold, London.

Edholm, O.G. and Weiner, J.S. (1981). Thermal physiology. In *The principles and practice of human physiology*, (ed. O.G. Edholm, J.S. Weiner), Chapter 3. Academic Press, London, NY.

Girardier, L. and Stock, M.J. (ed.) (1983). *Mammalian thermogenesis*. Chapman & Hall, London, NY.

Keatinge, W.R. (1969). *Survival in cold water*. Blackwell, Oxford.

Moran, E.F. (1979). *Human adaptability: an introduction to ecological anthropology*. Duxbury Press, MA.

7

Life at altitude

7.1 Introduction

Life at altitude is associated with a number of stressors of human physiology.

1. At a given latitude, it is generally colder at altitude than at sea-level. On average, every 150 m of ascent is associated with a 1°C fall in ambient temperature. Not only is the absolute air temperature lower in mountainous regions, but also wind speeds are often high so that there is, in addition, an appreciable 'wind chill factor' (see Chapter 6). Thus, ascent to altitude may impose considerable thermoregulatory demands on the body.

2. The relative humidity of the air decreases with increasing altitude. As a result there is increased insensible water loss by evaporation from the skin and in the breath. These losses are amplified by the increased wind velocities (see above) and the increased minute ventilation (see later) associated with life at altitude. Thus, at altitude, the dangers of dehydration must be opposed.

3. Although air temperature at altitude is lower than at sea-level, in the absence of cloud cover there is increased exposure to solar radiation, so that radiated heat gains may be higher. This exposure to solar radiation is further increased by reflection from any snow covering the ground. As solar radiation increases, so does ultraviolet radiation. The fact that prolonged exposure to ultraviolet radiation may lead to skin cancer is now well established.

To a large extent these problems can be avoided by behavioural changes, such as the use of appropriate clothing. However, there is a further major problem associated with life at altitude which cannot be avoided—the hypobaric environment. Since air is compressible, barometric pressure decreases exponentially as altitude increases and is approximately halved for each 5450 m of ascent (Fig. 7.1). Because the proportion of the atmosphere which is oxygen is constant at 20.93 per cent, the decrease in barometric pressure at altitude is paralleled by a decrease in ambient PO_2. As a result, alveolar and arterial PO_2 fall, resulting in a form of hypoxic hypoxia termed hypobaric hypoxia. The decrease in alveolar and, hence, arterial, PO_2 is greater than the decrease in ambient PO_2. This is because inspired air is always saturated with water vapour which exerts a pressure of 47 mmHg (6.4 kPa). Thus at an altitude of 5450 m, where ambient pressure is only approximately half the normal 760 mmHg at sea-level, the PO_2 of moist inspired gas is $(380-47) \times 0.2093 = 70$ mmHg (9.3 kPa). At the summit of Mount Everest (altitude 8848 m, barometric pressure approximately 253 mmHg), the inspired PO_2 is only 43 mmHg (5.7 kPa) (Fig. 7.1).

In spite of the hypoxic conditions, approximately 25 million people permanently inhabit regions above 3000 m and approximately 10 million above 4000 m. The highest known permanent residence is a mining community on Aucanquilcha (5950 m) in the Andes. In addition, an ever-increasing number of people expose themselves temporarily to hypoxic conditions, for example, during skiing holidays and, more recently, trekking holidays in remote mountainous regions as well as during serious mountaineering expeditions. With prolonged exposure to hypobaric conditions a number of physiological changes occur which allow an individual to acclimatize to the hypoxic environment. This chapter will concentrate on these changes. However, it is important to note first the adverse effects which can result if there is rapid exposure to altitude.

7.2 The effects of rapid exposure to altitude

Each year many millions of people are potentially exposed to extreme altitudes during air travel. Modern aircraft fly at an altitude of approx-

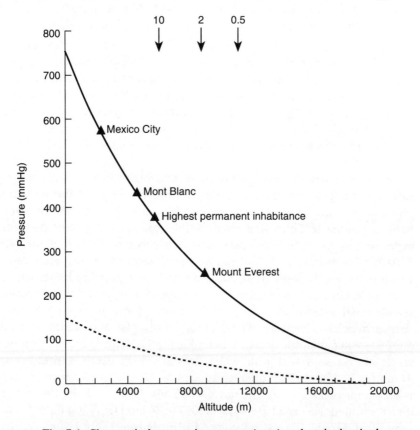

Fig. 7.1. Changes in barometric pressure (——) and moist inspired PO_2 (······), with increasing altitude. Numbers at the top indicate the time (min) of useful consciousness with sudden, immediate exposure to different altitudes.

imately 10 km (Concorde and some military aircraft approximately double this altitude). Passengers are not exposed to these extreme hypoxic conditions because the cabin is usually maintained at a pressure equivalent to an altitude of approximately 1900–2500 m. (The fact that aircraft are not pressurized to normal sea-level pressures, means that passengers are exposed to a mildly hypoxic environment. This indicates that those with marked cardiorespiratory problems, where there might be a pre-existing arterial hypoxia, should seek a doctor's advice before contemplating air travel.) However, should the pressurization system fail and there is a rapid decompression, the hypoxia is so severe as to cause unconsciousness and death. Thus, at an altitude of 10 km the time of useful consciousness with rapid decompression is approximately 45 s (grab that oxygen mask quickly!). A further consequence is a decompression sickness similar to that experienced by the deep sea diver (see Chapter 8).

Even rapid exposure to the altitudes found in mountainous regions can have marked adverse effects. For healthy individuals with no preexisting arterial hypoxia, no adverse effects have been noted below an altitude of 2500 m (see above). However, on rapid exposure to altitudes in the range 3000–6000 m, the symptoms associated with acute mountain sickness usually appear (see later). At altitudes above 4000 m the hypoxia causes cerebral hypoxia: there is usually progressive impairment of psychomotor performance with deterioration of sensory acuity, vigilance, judgement, speed of response, and manual dexterity. Above 6000 m consciousness is lost within a few minutes or within seconds at extreme altitude.

The symptoms of the acute mountain sickness seen at moderate altitudes usually disappear after a few days. If ascent to altitude is sufficiently slow, the cerebral hypoxia found at higher altitudes can be largely avoided, although mild cerebral signs are always seen in the lowland visitor at altitudes above 6000 m. However, the cerebral hypoxia is not so severe as to prevent mountaineers reaching the summit of Mount Everest without the use of supplementary oxygen. These facts indicate that, if the rate of ascent is gradual, physiological changes can occur which prevent many of the adverse effects and compensate for the hypoxic conditions. The way in which we can acclimatize to the hypoxic conditions found in mountainous regions, will now be described.

7.3 Acclimatization to altitude

7.3.1 Normal oxygen transport

Aerobic metabolism is dependent upon delivery of oxygen to the mitochondria. This takes place in four steps:

(1) alveolar ventilation—oxygen passing from the atmosphere to the alveoli;

(2) pulmonary oxygen diffusion—oxygen passing from the alveoli to the pulmonary capillary blood;

(3) transport of oxygen in the blood, bound to haemoglobin, from pulmonary to systemic capillaries; and

(4) tissue diffusion—the diffusion of oxygen from systemic capillary blood to the mitochondria in cells.

As shown in Fig. 7.2, a decrease in PO_2 occurs at each of these stages of oxygen transport. Thus, oxygen can be thought of as passing down a cascade of partial pressure from atmosphere to tissues, there being a total

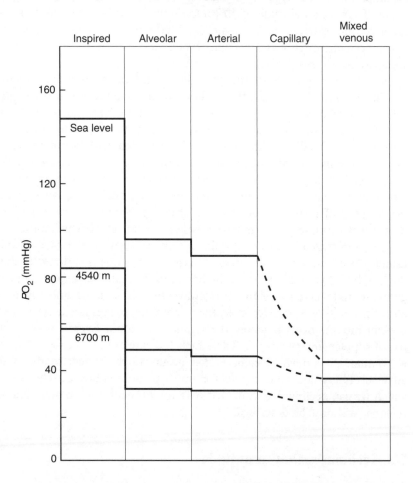

Fig. 7.2. Mean PO_2s in the oxygen cascade from inspired air to mixed venous blood. PO_2s are shown in three groups of subjects: sea-level native, subjects native to 4540 m, and climbers at 6700 m. From Heath, D., and Williams, D.R. (1981). *Man at high altitude*, 2nd edn. Churchill Livingstone, Edinburgh. Reprinted by permission of Butterworth-Heinemann Ltd.

pressure gradient from inspired air to mixed venous blood of approximately 110 mmHg (14.6 kPa). It is obvious from Fig. 7.2 that if the slope of this cascade did not change, then at an altitude of 4540 m (inspired $PO_2 = 82$ mmHg), this same gradient would result in a mixed venous PO_2 of approximately -30 mmHg! However, as indicated in Fig. 7.2, acclimatization to altitude involves a decrease in slope of the oxygen cascade such that the mixed venous PO_2 is little changed. Such acclimatization may be achieved by modifying each of the four steps involved in oxygen transport.

Before describing these modifications it is important to note from the outset that the modifications seen in a normal person living at sea-level (low altitude native, LAN) who visits altitude may be qualitatively and quantitatively different in the first few hours or days of exposure from those after several weeks or months at altitude. Furthermore, the acclimatization seen in the longer term visitor is often different from the 'acquired acclimatization' seen in a person born and bred at altitude (high altitude native, HAN). There is little evidence of adaptation in the human HAN ('adaptation' is used here in its pure Darwinian definition as changes which are inherited).

7.3.2 Pulmonary ventilation

Figure 7.2 shows that in both the LAN visitor and the HAN, the main change decreasing the slope of the oxygen cascade is a reduction in the PO_2 difference between inspired and alveolar air. This is caused by an increase in minute ventilation (hyperventilation).

Hyperventilation is seen in the newly arrived visitor to altitude, but only at altitudes in excess of 3000 m (this corresponds to the altitude at which alveolar PO_2 (P_AO_2) falls to 65 mmHg). At 3000 m hyperventilation is slight, but increases progressively with increasing altitude, reaching a maximum at approximately 6000 m, where minute ventilation exceeds that at sea-level by 65 per cent (Fig. 7.3).

This initial hyperventilation is entirely due to stimulation of the peripheral chemoreceptors of the carotid and aortic bodies by the fall in arterial PO_2 (P_aO_2). Thus, it rapidly ceases if the visitor returns to sea-level or is given 100 per cent oxygen to breathe and is absent in individuals in whom the arterial chemoreceptors have been denervated.

The adaptive value of this hyperventilation is that it increases alveolar ventilation and, hence, reduces the fall in P_AO_2 and P_aO_2. However, there is also a disadvantage; hyperventilation causes an increased loss of carbon dioxide such that P_ACO_2 and P_aCO_2 fall (Fig. 7.4). As would be predicted from the Henderson–Hasselbach equation for the bicarbonate buffer system, this causes a respiratory alkalosis and arterial pH rises (Fig. 7.4). The fall in P_aCO_2 also leads to a fall in the PCO_2 of cerebrospinal fluid (CSF) and its pH rises as well. This alkalosis in the region of the central, medullary chemoreceptors tends to inhibit ventilation (it should be recalled that the central chemoreceptors and, hence, ventilation are stimulated by an increase in H$^+$ concentration (decrease in pH) of their immediate environment). Thus, on initial exposure to hypoxic conditions there are competing influences on minute ventilation—the fall in P_aO_2 stimulating ventilation and the fall in P_aCO_2, via changes in H$^+$ concentration of the CSF, inhibiting it. This explains why the increase in ventilation on first exposure to altitude is modest and is absent below altitudes of 3000 m. That is, until P_aO_2 falls to approximately 60 mmHg (8 kPa) (the P_aO_2 found initially at an altitude of 3000 m), the hypoxic drive to ventilation from the peripheral chemoreceptors is overcome completely by the inhibition of the central chemoreceptors, so that no change in ventilation occurs. At altitudes above 3000 m, the drive to ventilation from the peripheral chemoreceptors is greater than the brake from the central chemoreceptors, so ventilation rises. Even so, the ventilation is not as great as it would be if the development of alkalosis was prevented.

If the LAN visitor remains at altitude, minute ventilation (and, hence, P_aO_2) continues to increase for several days (Figs 7.3 and 7.4). Unlike the initial phase of hyperventilation, this phase develops at altitudes below 3000 m (Fig. 7.3). The time taken for this secondary rise in ventilation to

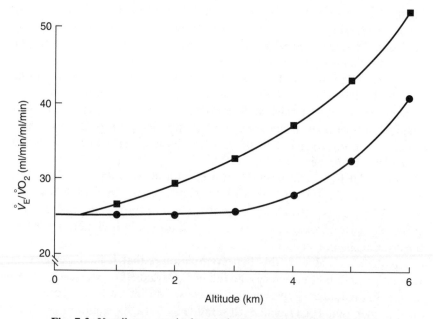

Fig. 7.3. Ventilatory equivalent (minute ventilation/rate of oxygen consumption, $\dot{V}_E/\dot{V}O_2$) at different altitudes in sea-level subjects acutely exposed to altitude (●——●) and after 4 days acclimatization (■——■). From Lenfant, C. and Sullivan, K. (1971). Reprinted by permission of *The New England Journal of Medicine*, **294**, 1298–1309.

reach its maximum increases with increasing altitude; at 3000–4000 m it usually takes approximately 1–2 weeks. Once this secondary rise in ventilation has developed it persists as long as the visitor stays at altitude and continues for some time even if the visitor breathes oxygen to return their P_aO_2 back to sea-level values. Thus, when the visitor returns to sea-level there is a period of deacclimatization.

The mechanism of the secondary rise in ventilation seen in the visitor has not been clearly resolved. The rise in ventilation decreases the P_aCO_2 further, which would be expected to worsen the respiratory alkalosis and depress ventilation. With time the arterial respiratory alkalosis is compensated for by renal excretion of HCO_3^-, so that the blood buffer base is decreased. In the long-term such compensation must account, in part, for the secondary rise. However, even when compensated by renal mechanisms,

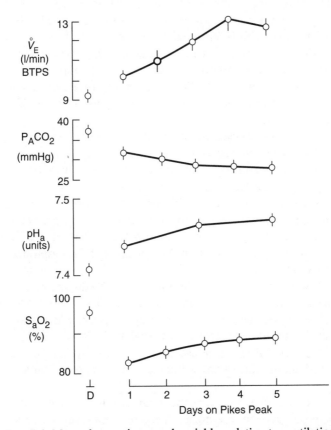

Fig. 7.4. Mean changes in several variables relating to ventilation in subjects at Denver (D), 1600 m and during the first 5 days at an altitude of 4300 m on Pikes Peak. S_aO_2, saturation of arterial blood with oxygen. From Huang, S.Y., Alexander, J.K., Grover, R.F., Maher, J.T., McCullough, R.E., McCullough, R.G., Moore, L.G., *et al.* (1984). *Journal of Applied Physiology*, **56**, 602–4.

arterial pH is not returned to normal; there is still a slight arterial alkalosis. Furthermore, the time course of renal compensation is too slow to account for the rate at which ventilation rises. This indicates that other mechanisms are involved.

The problems of assessing the control mechanisms involved become apparent when it is recalled that the precise site of the medullary chemoreceptors is unknown and whether they respond directly to the pH of the CSF or the pH of the brain interstitial fluid has not been resolved. One early explanation of the secondary rise in ventilation suggested that the pH of the CSF was rapidly returned to normal by active transport of HCO_3^- out of the CSF by the choroid plexus. Alternatively, the hypoxia at altitude may lead to increased anaerobic metabolism by the brain resulting in increased lactate production (and, hence, H^+). Again, this would tend to correct the alkalosis of the CSF. However, measurements of the pH of the CSF in acclimatized subjects have not always confirmed the return of pH of the CSF to normal, the pH remaining slightly elevated compared with the values found at sea-level. More recently it has been suggested that the secondary rise in ventilation results from 'central sensitization' of respiratory centres to peripheral chemoreceptor inputs but, in addition, there may be sensitization of peripheral chemoreceptors with chronic hypoxia, a finding recently demonstrated in rats.

Whatever the mechanisms involved, the respiratory system behaves as though it has been reset to run at a lower P_aCO_2. The carbon dioxide response curve (the approximately linear increase in ventilation with increasing P_aCO_2) is shifted to the left to a lower intercept (the hypothetical PCO_2 at which ventilation would be zero). Furthermore, the slope of the curve is increased so that a given rise in PCO_2 results in a greater increase in ventilation. Overall, once acclimatization has occurred the respiratory system is more sensitive to carbon dioxide so that the respiratory centres respond to a lower PCO_2.

An increase in ventilation to altitude is undoubtedly the most important of the various responses involved in acclimatization of the LAN visitor to altitude. This importance can be seen from Fig. 7.2, which shows that in climbers acclimatized to an altitude of 6700 m, P_AO_2 is 30 mmHg (4 kPa). Without any ventilatory response and assuming no change in carbon dioxide production, the value would have been approximately 9 mmHg (1.2 kPa).

Like the acclimatized visitor, the high altitude native (HAN) hyperventilates in comparison to a normal person at sea-level. However, studies of HANs of the Himalayas and Andes have shown that their ventilation is approximately 20 per cent less than in acclimatized visitors. At first sight it might appear as though the HAN is less well acclimatized to the hypoxic conditions. However, this relative decrease in ventilation is probably adaptive (in so far as reduced pulmonary work decreases energy and, hence, oxygen demands), the HAN using less energy-consuming methods to compensate for the hypoxic conditions (for example, more efficient pulmonary gas exchange, see below).

The acclimatized visitor and the HAN also differ in their response to hypoxia. Whereas the acclimatized visitor still shows an increased ventilation when acutely exposed to low PO_2, the HAN shows little change in ventilation over a wide range of inspired PO_2, although a very low P_AO_2 (<30 mmHg) still induces an increase in ventilation. This blunted hypoxic response persists in HANs even after they have lived for several years at sealevel. However, it is not a form of adaptation (that is, genetically determined). The same blunting develops in individuals of sea-level ancestry born at altitude or taken there during early infancy and it occurs in those who have a chronic arterial hypoxia due to congenital heart defect during infancy. These findings indicate that the blunted hypoxia is acquired with chronic hypoxia during early childhood. The mechanism responsible for blunting has not been resolved, but is thought to be associated with several histological and biochemical changes and hypertrophy found in the carotid bodies of the HAN.

The cause of the hyperventilation seen in the HAN in spite of a blunted hypoxic response is also uncertain. The pH of the CSF in the HAN is generally similar to, or only very slightly acidic compared with those of the LAN. Thus, the 'setting' of the central chemoreceptors is probably close to that normally found at sea-level and so cannot account for the hyperventilation seen in the HAN.

7.3.3 Pulmonary oxygen transfer

Clearly the increased ventilation seen at altitude increases P_AO_2 and, thus, the driving pressure for oxygen transfer to the pulmonary capillary blood. Further advantage would be gained if the pulmonary oxygen diffusing capacity were increased (that is, if a given oxygen uptake required a smaller $P_AO_2 - P_aO_2$ difference). Such an increase in diffusing capacity can be achieved by an increase in alveolar surface area in contact with functioning pulmonary capillaries. An increased diffusing capacity can also be achieved by minimizing ventilation/perfusion inequalities, increasing pulmonary blood volume, and increasing haemoglobin concentration. The size of the $P_AO_2 - P_aO_2$ difference may also be significant. Normally in healthy individuals at sea-level the $P_AO_2 - P_aO_2$ difference is 5–15 mmHg. With a reduced P_AO_2, as seen at altitude, such a difference might lead to the steep portion of the oxyhaemoglobin dissociation curve being approached and, thus, a large fall in the quantity of oxygen carried bound to haemoglobin.

There is no evidence to indicate significant changes in pulmonary diffusing capacity in the short-term visitor. This leads to a significant fall in arterial oxygen saturation during exercise (see later). In contrast, pulmonary diffusing capacity in the HAN is greater at rest by some 20–30 per cent, resulting in a much reduced $P_AO_2 - P_aO_2$ gradient. There are also reports of increased diffusing capacity of LANs who have remained at altitude for several years.

The increased pulmonary diffusing capacity in the HAN is probably due largely to an increased alveolar surface area. Thus, a characteristic of some HANs of the Andes is a barrel-shaped chest and increased lung volumes, especially residual volume. Morphometric measurements of the lungs of HANs at 3840 m have shown alveoli which are larger and greater in number than those of LANs of the same stature.

Increases in pulmonary blood volume have been reported in HANs which will also lead to an increased diffusing capacity. In addition, it is likely that the increase in pulmonary arterial pressure seen in HANs (see later) leads to an opening of a larger number of pulmonary capillaries (those in the apices of the lungs). However, studies of the ventilation/perfusion ratio in HANs have shown inconsistent changes.

7.3.4 Blood oxygen transport

The rate at which oxygen is transported from the lungs to tissues is determined by the product cardiac output × haemoglobin concentration ([Hb]) × arterial saturation of haemoglobin with oxygen (S_aO_2).

7.3.4.1 *Haemoglobin concentrations at altitudes*

Both the visitor and the HAN show an increase in erythrocyte count (polycythaemia). As a result [Hb] rises, although a small proportion of the rise is accounted for by a small fall in plasma volume resulting in haemo-concentration.

The polycythaemic response increases linearly up to approximately 3700 m, but thereafter rises more rapidly with increasing altitude. Table 7.1 shows some mean haematological findings in a group of mountaineers and a group of HANs, as well as normal values found at sea-level.

The polycythaemic response is due to increased secretion of erythro-poietin resulting from the decreased P_aO_2 sensed by the kidneys. Plasma erythropoietin concentration rises within the first 2 hours of altitude exposure and reaches a maximum within a day. Thereafter, erythropoietin secretion falls somewhat as the P_aO_2 improves with the hyperventilation and other mechanisms of acclimatization. Because of the lag between erythropoietin secretion and red cell production, red cell count does not start to rise until approximately 3–5 days of altitude exposure. The full erythropoietic response may then take several weeks to develop.

The increase in [Hb] greatly increases the oxygen carrying capacity of blood. With the fall in P_aO_2 at altitude the S_aO_2 also falls (see Fig. 7.4) but the rise in [Hb] ensures that arterial oxygen **content** is maintained at or even

Table 7.1. Haematological values in Everest mountaineers at 5790 m, inhabitants of Morococha in the Andes (4540 m) and normal values at sea-level

	Rbc count ($\times 10^{12}$/litre)	Haematocrit (%)	Hb concentration (g/d litre)
Sea-level	5.0	45.0	14.8
4540 m	6.4	59.5	20.1
5790 m	5.6	55.8	19.6

All values are for male subjects.

above the value at sea-level. If, however, S_aO_2 falls below 70 per cent, the arterial oxygen content starts to decline.

The benefit gained from the erythropoietic response seems obvious. However, recently this benefit has been questioned. This is because, as haematocrit rises, so does the viscosity of blood. In turn, this tends to decrease blood flow and increase the work of the heart. Mathematical modelling has shown that the 'optimal haematocrit' is close to that normally found at sea-level. Thus, many now believe that the polycythaemia found at altitude is not as helpful as once was thought. This view is supported by the observation that in mammalian species genetically **adapted** to altitude, such as the South American camelids (llama and alpaca), there is little or no increase in haematocrit.

7.3.4.2 *Changes in cardiac output and the systemic circulation*

Studies of changes in resting cardiac output in visitors during the first few hours and days of altitude exposure have not given consistent results. All agree that there is an increase in heart rate, but while some have found no change in stroke volume and, thus, an elevated cardiac output (Fig. 7.5), others have found a diminished stroke volume and unchanged cardiac output. However, all studies agree that after several days, cardiac output at rest is equal to or slightly below that at sea-level, although heart rate remains elevated and, thus, stroke volume is decreased (Fig. 7.5). This conclusion is valid up to altitudes of 7100 m in the acclimatized mountaineer, although with increasing altitude there is a gradual increase in heart rate and proportional decrease in stroke volume.

The tachycardia found at altitude appears to be due to a generalized increase in sympathetic activity, as evidenced by raised plasma and urinary catecholamine concentrations. The cause of the diminished stroke volume is less clearly understood. Originally it was thought that hypoxia directly caused a fall in myocardial contractility. However, recent results from mountaineers at high altitude have indicated that myocardial contractility is maintained and suggest that the decreased stroke volume is caused by decreased right atrial filling.

Like the acclimatized visitor, the HAN also shows a resting cardiac output similar to that normally found at sea-level, but in this case heart rate and stroke volume are normal. An increase in cardiac output might be expected in so far as it would increase oxygen delivery to the tissues. However, such an increase would involve extra myocardial oxygen consumption and, thus, offset the advantage gained. Instead, the oxygen demands of the tissues are met by greater extraction of oxygen rather than increasing blood flow.

Although resting cardiac output is largely unaltered at altitude, there is a redistribution of blood flow so that the vital organs receive a larger proportion of the cardiac output than at sea-level. Thus, for example, blood flow is distributed away from the gut and skin. Renal blood flow is also decreased in the HAN but there is only a small fall in glomerular filtration rate due to an increased filtration fraction.

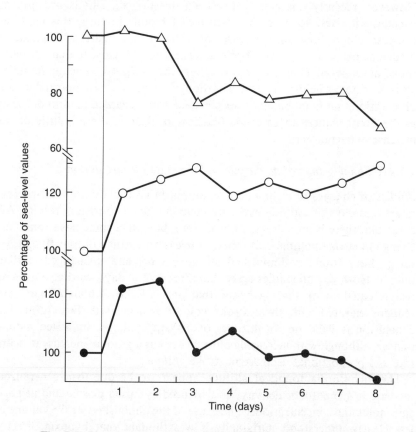

Fig. 7.5. Changes in cardiac output (●——●), stroke volume (△——△) and heart rate (○——○), in three subjects during the first 8 days exposure to an altitude of 3800 m, expressed as percentage of sea-level values. Data of Klausen, K. (1966). *Journal of Applied Physiology*, **21**, 609–16.

On first exposure to altitude, an increase in coronary blood flow is found in the visitor, a result expected from the classical vasodilator action of hypoxia at altitude. However, in one study, after 10 days at an altitude of 3100 m, the visitors' coronary blood flow fell by 30 per cent but oxygen uptake by the myocardium was largely maintained by a 28 per cent increase in oxygen extraction. In the HAN, coronary blood flow has also been reported to be diminished by 30 per cent but, at least in part, this is compensated by an increased vascularization of the myocardium.

Although at rest the cardiac output of the visitor acclimatized to altitude is little different from that found normally at sea-level, during maximal exercise the maximum cardiac output achieved is reduced. This is due to a decreased maximum stroke volume and, in some studies, a small fall in maximum heart rate achieved. However, it is not clear whether this fall in maximum cardiac output is the cause of the low maximum aerobic work capacities found in the visitor (see later) or is a result of the reduced maximal work capacity and, hence, reduced maximum oxygen consumption. By contrast, the HAN is generally able to achieve maximal cardiac outputs similar to those of people of similar physical ability at sea-level.

7.3.4.3 *Haemoglobin affinity for oxygen*

The saturation of haemoglobin with oxygen is determined by the PO_2, as described by the oxyhaemoglobin (O_2–Hb) dissociation curve. The saturation of haemoglobin at any given PO_2 is also affected by its affinity for oxygen. Changes in the affinity of haemoglobin are reflected in a change in the position and shape of the O_2–Hb curve and are investigated by measuring the P_{50}. The P_{50} is the PO_2 giving 50 per cent saturation of haemoglobin and is frequently measured under standard conditions, namely 37°C and pH 7.4. Under such conditions at sea-level it is usually in the range 26–28 mmHg (3.4–3.7 kPa).

Many studies have indicated that in both the acclimatized visitor and the HAN at altitude there is a rise in P_{50} (rightward shift of the O_2–Hb curve). In one study, P_{50} in normal subjects rose from 26.6 (3.6) to 28.6 mmHg (3.8 kPa) within 12 h of their being transported to 4530 m and rose further to 31 mmHg (4.1 kPa) after 3 days at this altitude. HANs at the same altitude had a P_{50} of 30.7 mmHg (4.1 kPa). Such a rightward shift of the O_2–Hb curve can be considered advantageous in that it aids the unloading of oxygen from blood in the tissues. That is, a rightward shift of the O_2–Hb curve ensures a greater desaturation of haemoglobin (release of oxygen) for any given PO_2 and, thus, maintains an adequate capillary PO_2 for tissue oxygen diffusion.

The increase in P_{50} has been attributed to an increased concentration of 2,3-diphosphoglycerate (2,3-DPG) within erythrocytes which is induced, at least in part, by the respiratory alkalosis. By binding to the β-chains of the haemoglobin molecule, 2,3-DPG favours the stabilization of the deoxy form of haemoglobin so that unloading of oxygen is facilitated. Increases in 2,3-DPG concentrations are found in both the HAN and in the visitor to altitude, in the latter case within 15 h of exposure to altitude. The concentration of 2,3-DPG increases progressively up to an altitude of approximately 4500 m, above which no further increases have been observed.

Recently the advantage gained by an increased P_{50} has been questioned because, although this aids the unloading of oxygen from blood at the tissues, it hinders loading of blood with oxygen at the lungs. Furthermore, the accuracy of the measured increase in P_{50} at altitude has been questioned. This is because in many studies of haemoglobin affinity, the P_{50} has been measured under standard conditions (pH 7.4). But many studies have indicated that the respiratory alkalosis which develops at altitude is not fully compensated for, so that blood remains slightly alkaline. This would cause a decrease in P_{50} (leftward shift of the O_2–Hb curve). Thus, several recent studies, in which *in vivo* P_{50} was measured, have found no change of P_{50} in both visitors and HANs above altitudes of 3000 m. That is, the leftward shift of the O_2–Hb curve due to an increased pH offsets the rightward shift caused by 2,3-DPG; when a marked alkalosis develops, a net leftward shift may be found. Thus, shifts in the position of the O_2–Hb curve are probably of less significance in the process of acclimatization to altitude than was previously thought.

It is interesting to note that a leftward shift of the O_2–Hb curve is often found in many mammals **adapted** to altitude, indicating that natural selection seems to favour a high O_2–Hb affinity in a hypoxic environment. There is some evidence to indicate an advantage to be gained by a leftward shift of the O_2–Hb curve in humans too. Thus,

(1) in the human fetus, which has a P_aO_2 equivalent to that in mountaineers breathing air near the summit of Mount Everest, the O_2–Hb curve is shifted to the left (see Chapter 2);

(2) when two subjects possessing a mutant haemoglobin with a high oxygen affinity were transported to an altitude of 3100 m, no decrement in maximal oxygen consumption during maximal exercise was found, although such a decrement was found in their normal siblings.

7.3.5 Tissue diffusion and usage of oxygen

Movement of oxygen from capillary blood to mitochondria occurs by simple diffusion. As characterized by the Fick equation, the rate of this diffusion is determined by the PO_2 gradient and by the distance and surface area over which diffusion occurs. Thus, it has long been argued that increased capillarization of the tissues will occur at altitude so as to aid oxygen diffusion to the tissues by decreasing the diffusion distance. Indeed, an increased density of functional capillaries has been observed in several mammalian species acclimatized to altitude, especially in the cerebral cortex, myocardium, and skeletal muscle, although it is not clear whether this results from formation of new capillaries or the opening up of pre-existing ones. However, it is not universally accepted that the increased capillary density **results** from chronic hypoxia. This is because hypoxic exposure in animals is often accompanied by a decrease in body weight. There is a linear relationship between muscle fibre cross-sectional area and body weight and an inverse relationship between capillary density and muscle fibre cross-sectional area. Thus, with decreased body weight there is an increased capillary density.

Studies of tissue capillarization in humans have understandably been less frequent. None the less, recent studies on acclimatized Himalayan climbers and Sherpas have shown an increased capillary density and decreased muscle fibre cross-sectional area in skeletal muscle, resulting in a shortened diffusion path for oxygen.

Oxygen is useful only if it enters the mitochondria. Thus, there has been considerable interest in whether or not the volume density of mitochondria and their distribution in the cell is altered by chronic hypoxia. In the study on Sherpas and acclimatized climbers referred to above, there was a **decrease** in skeletal muscle mitochondrial volume density. Similarly, many studies of altitude-adapted animals have failed to show changes in the density or distribution of mitochondria within the cell.

In both altitude-adapted mammals and HANs an increased skeletal muscle concentration of myoglobin has been observed. This would not only increase oxygen reserves for periods of exercise but also facilitate the diffusion of oxygen through the myoplasm.

7.4 Limits of acclimatization—life at extreme altitudes

The highest permanent inhabitants are the miners on the mountain Aucanquilcha (5950 m) in Chile. These miners work at an altitude of 5790 m but live at an altitude of 5390 m which appears to be the limit for 'complete adjustment'. They refuse to live permanently at the work site due to difficulty in sleeping. Similarly mountaineers often report 'high altitude deterioration', a progressive deterioration of mental and physical condition, at altitudes in excess of 5800 m.

However, we can survive for short periods at altitudes in excess of this. Indeed, the summit of Mount Everest (8848 m) has been conquered without the need for supplemental oxygen but this appears to be the limit to human endurance. Thus, Messner, the first to reach the summit without supplemental oxygen, said "I am nothing more than a single, narrow, gasping lung . . .".

Over the last decade two studies have greatly increased our knowledge of physiological responses that occur when man ascends to extreme altitudes. The first, in 1981, was the American Medical Research Expedition to Everest (ARMEE) in which studies were made of mountaineers at 5400 and 6400 m and some measurements were made on the summit. The other was Operation Everest II in which eight volunteers simulated a gradual ascent over 40 days to the summit of Mount Everest in a low pressure chamber. These studies show the marked changes that occur. Thus, at the summit, although

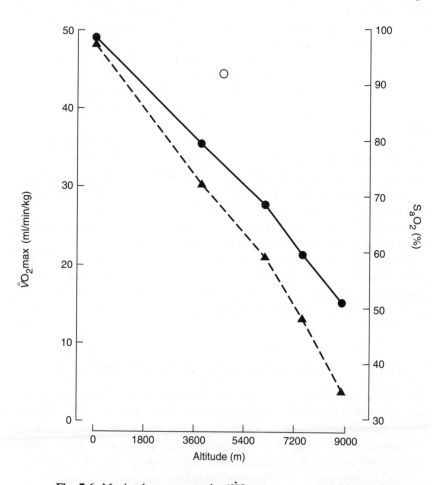

Fig. 7.6. Maximal oxygen uptake ($\dot{V}O_2$max, ●——●), and arterial oxygen saturation (S_aO_2, ▲------▲) in five subjects studied at different simulated altitudes. Data of Cymerman, A., Reeves, J.T., Sutton, J.R., Rock, P.B., Groves, B.M., Malconian, M.K., *et al.* (1989). *Journal of Applied Physiology*, **66**, 2446–53. ○, maximal oxygen uptake in a highland native at 4540 m.

inspired PO_2 was 42 mmHg (5.6 kPa), P_AO_2 was maintained at approximately 35 mmHg (4.7 kPa) by a four-fold increase in alveolar ventilation. The mean P_aO_2 at rest was 30 mmHg (4.0 kPa) and P_aCO_2 was 12 mmHg (1.6 kPa). (At sea-level the corresponding values for these subjects were 95 and 35 mmHg respectively.) There was also a marked respiratory alkalosis (pH 7.56) and, as a result, a leftward shift of the O_2–Hb curve (P_{50} approximately 24 mmHg). Arterial saturation of haemoglobin with oxygen (S_aO_2) was 60 per cent. On exercise, maximal oxygen consumption was only 28 per cent of the value attained by the subjects at sea-level and P_aO_2 and S_aO_2 decreased further (28 mmHg and 35 per cent respectively) (see also Fig. 7.6).

Cardiac function appeared to be maintained, with a normal relationshp between cardiac output and oxygen consumption. That is, for a given work rate, the cardiac output was the same as at sea-level, although, of course, maximal work rates (and, therefore, cardiac outputs) were decreased. However, at a given cardiac output, heart rate was increased and stroke volume correspondingly reduced.

At these high altitudes, short- and long-term memory declined and manual dexterity decreased. Interestingly, there seemed to be some residual impairment in CNS function even on return to sea-level, which persisted for at least 1 year. It appears that in such markedly hypoxic conditions, the CNS did not escape completely unscathed.

A major conclusion from both studies was that the main adaptive process which allowed ascent to these extreme altitudes was the increase in ventilation: those who made it to the summit were those who showed the greatest hypoxic ventilatory response at sea-level.

7.5 Work performance at altitude

The foregoing sections have described the physiological changes which occur during acclimatization to chronic hypoxia. At rest these changes maintain sufficient oxygen delivery in order to prevent the cerebral effects seen with acute rapid hypoxia, at least up to an altitude of approximately 6000 m. This is not the case during exercise, when the feeling of comfort rapidly disappears as ventilation and breathlessness increase. Not surprisingly, work capacity, as assessed by the maximum attainable rate of oxygen consumption ($\dot{V}O_2$max), is reduced in the visitor to altitude. This reduction is most marked during the first few days but is attenuated as acclimatization takes place. However, even after several months at altitude, $\dot{V}O_2$max never achieves the value obtained by the same individual at sea-level. As might be expected, the decrement in $\dot{V}O_2$max becomes greater with increasing altitude (Fig. 7.6).

During exercise at altitude the normal linear relationship between cardiac output and oxygen consumption is maintained, but maximal cardiac outputs are decreased. It is not clear whether this decrease is responsible, in part, for the decrease in $\dot{V}O_2$max or results from the lowered $\dot{V}O_2$max. The maximum minute ventilation achieved at $\dot{V}O_2$max is unaltered from that achieved at sea-level but, at a given work load, minute ventilation is higher. A major factor which seems to limit exercise performance is diffusion limitation across the alveolar–capillary membranes. Thus, with increasing altitude, there is a progressive fall in S_aO_2 during exercise (Fig. 7.6).

By contrast with the acclimatized visitor, the HAN has a $\dot{V}O_2$max which, at least up to approximately 4500 m, is similar to or only slightly decreased from that found in individuals of similar athletic training at sea-level. Thus, it has long been recognized, for example, that the Sherpas of the high Himalayas are able to carry larger loads for longer periods than the mountaineers who employ them, indeed, the ego of the male mountaineers is not boosted when it is found that the Sherpanis (Sherpa women) are able to carry larger loads than they.

The physiological changes which give the HAN this greater work capacity have not been resolved. However, the fact that individuals of sea-level ancestry but reared at altitude develop a $\dot{V}O_2$max similar to that of the HAN indicates that developmental processes are involved rather than a genetic change.

During maximal exercise at altitude the rise in blood lactate concentration in the acclimatized visitor and the HAN is not as great as in maximal exercise at sea-level. In view of the hypoxic conditions at altitude, this is a rather unexpected result. In the HAN, but not in the visitor, this 'lactate paradox' persists even after 6 weeks at sea-level suggesting a developmental or genetic change. The decreased blood lactate appears to be due to decreased release of lactate by exercising muscle, rather than increased removal from blood, although the reason for this decreased release has not been resolved. The adaptive value of the decreased lactate production is considered to be the efficiency advantage (high ATP yield per mole of substrate used) of aerobic metabolism vs anaerobic glycolysis.

7.6 Adaptation versus acclimatization

Figure 7.7 summarizes the various physiological changes which compensate for the hypoxic conditions at altitude and thereby allow survival. It can be seen that whilst the changes are qualitatively the same in the lowland visitor and the HAN, quantitatively they may be different. These differences (larger diffusing capacity, lower minute ventilation, and increased $\dot{V}O_2$max) are also seen in LANs who migrate to altitude during early childhood, indicating that they are developmental rather than genetic in origin. This natural acclimatization unquestionably compensates more for the hypoxic conditions than the acclimatization acquired by the lowland visitor, as evidenced by the greater $\dot{V}O_2$max.

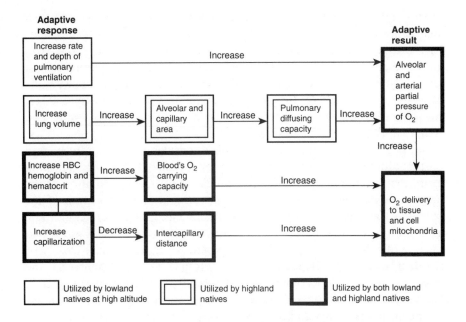

Fig. 7.7. The pathways involved in acclimatization to altitude in the highland and lowland native. From Frisancho, A.R. (1975). *Science*, **187**, 313–19. Reprinted by permission, Copyright (1975) by the AAAS.

It is interesting to note that many mammalian and avian species indigenous to mountain regions and which are believed to be genetically **adapted** to hypoxic conditions, often show different strategies for compensating for the hypoxic environment from those shown by acclimatized humans. For example, many do not show a polycythaemia or increased blood 2,3-DPG concentration. In addition, there is often little hyperventilation while a leftward shift of the O_2–Hb curve is the norm. Such animals compensate for the hypoxia by increasing the extraction of oxygen from blood at the tissues and by more efficient utilization of oxygen, in contrast to the decrease in the gradient of the 'oxygen cascade' from air to tissues seen in humans.

7.7 Other effects of chronic hypoxia

7.7.1 Pulmonary hypertension

It is well known that alveolar hypoxia induces vasoconstriction in the small arteries and arterioles of the pulmonary circulation, leading to an increase in pulmonary vascular resistance and, ultimately, to pulmonary arterial hypertension. Not surprisingly, therefore, some degree of pulmonary hypertension is found at altitude. In the short-term visitor it is small since the respiratory alkalosis which develops (see earlier) attenuates the response of the pulmonary arterioles to hypoxia. With increasing altitude and duration of stay, however, pulmonary vascular resistance rises further as persistent contraction of the small pulmonary arteries is associated with muscularization and constriction of pulmonary arterioles. Thus, in the long-term visitor to altitude and the HAN there is a mild pulmonary hypertension at rest which becomes more marked with exercise. For example, in one study of HANs in the Andes at 4540 m, mean pulmonary arterial pressure at rest was 28 mmHg (3.7 kPa) (cf. normal sea-level value, 15 mmHg) and rose to 60 mmHg (8.0 kPa) during exercise.

The degree of pulmonary hypertension is considerably greater in children born at altitude, at least up to the age of approximately 5 years. Following birth, the increase in P_aO_2 and P_AO_2 which results from ventilation of the lungs reverses the profound vasoconstriction and muscularization of the pulmonary arterial tree found during fetal life (see Chapter 2). At altitude, as a result of the lower ambient PO_2, the rise of P_AO_2 is not as great, and the rate of reversal correspondingly decreased. In addition, since closure of the ductus arteriosus depends upon the rising P_aO_2 (see Chapter 2), the lesser rise at altitude leads to a less powerful constriction of the ductus. Consequently, at altitude there is a greater incidence of patent ductus arteriosus in the young and this, by allowing some left to right shunt (that is, from aorta to pulmonary artery), accentuates the pulmonary hypertension.

7.7.2 Growth in the high altitude native

Children born at altitude are generally of low birth weight and are reduced in body size and growth rate at all postnatal ages. The reduced growth rate seems to be due, in part, to hypoxia *per se* but the generally poor nutritional status and socio-economic conditions often found in mountainous populations, are also thought to play a role.

The lungs are spared this reduction because growth of the lungs is stimulated by hypoxia. Thus, the HAN has a larger lung volume and vital capacity. The advantage gained from this larger lung volume, in terms of oxygen diffusing capacity, has already been described in an earlier section. The development of this larger lung volume does not seem to be a form of adaptation since children of sea-level ancestry raised at altitude also develop an increased lung capacity. By contrast, the larger chest dimensions found in several Andean populations seem to be under some genetic control since they are not found in other mountainous people who, none the less, still have increased lung volumes.

7.7.3 Maternal and fetal physiology

Even at sea-level the fetus is living on the brink in terms of oxygen availability, that is, the PO_2 of blood in the umbilical vein is approximately

30 mmHg (4 kPa) only (see Chapter 2). Such a low P_aO_2 is found in adult humans at an altitude equivalent to the summit of Mount Everest (see earlier). It might be predicted, therefore, that the fetus at altitude will suffer some degree of hypoxia. However, a comparison of humans at 4200 m and at sea-level reveals no significant differences in the PO_2 of blood from fetal scalps sampled at delivery. Similarly, in several mammalian species at altitude, fetal PO_2s similar to those normally found at sea-level have been recorded. Despite no obvious change in fetal PO_2, a slightly elevated haematocrit at term has been reported in infants born at 3700 and 4500 m, perhaps indicating some degree of fetal hypoxia. At worst this hypoxia can only be mild, indicating that there must be changes in maternal and/or placental physiology to compensate for the hypoxic environment.

Maternal hyperventilation and an increased haemoglobin concentration have been found during pregnancy in women at 3100 m, such that arterial oxygen content was as high as that in pregnant women at sea-level. The increase in minute ventilation was associated with an increased sensitivity to hypoxia which developed during pregnancy. In a study of Tibetan women at altitude, an increase in uterine arterial flow velocity, probably indicating an increase in uterine blood flow, was found. This increased flow, together with the improved arterial oxygen content described above, will increase oxygen delivery to the fetus. In addition, there appear to be several changes in placental morphology, including increased vascularity, which indicate a shortening of the diffusion distances and reduction in the oxygen diffusion gradient between mother and fetus.

7.7.4 Endocrine changes

The hypoxia associated with ascent to altitude induces the secretion of the stress hormones, adrenal glucocorticoids, and catecholamines. The major increases in plasma concentrations of these hormones occur during the first week at altitude. Thereafter, concentrations have usually been found to fall towards normal. However, in a recent study of HANs at 3700 m, a slightly hyperplastic adrenal cortex was found together with an increased population of corticotrophs in the anterior pituitary. It was suggested that greater amounts of ACTH were required to maintain normal adrenocortical function under hypoxic conditions.

Studies of experimental animals at high altitudes have usually indicated a depression of thyroid function. However, in a recent study of humans, increased thyroxine (T_4) and tri-iodothyronine (T_3) levels were found in visitors during a 3 week stay at 3500 m. Long-term visitors and HANs at this altitude also had elevated plasma T_4 and T_3 concentrations which were greater than those of the short-term visitors. Neither plasma TSH nor thyroid-binding globulin concentrations were significantly different from those normally found at sea-level.

Several hormones associated with body fluid homeostasis are also affected by altitude. The increased red cell count and blood volume associated with acclimatization to altitude, result in a decreased secretion of aldosterone and vasopressin (ADH). Thus, a natriuresis and diuresis often develop. However, in those individuals who seem to be more susceptible to acute mountain sickness (see below), a decrease in urine flow and fluid retention may develop on first exposure to altitude. Inconsistent changes in atrial natriuretic peptide (ANP) concentrations in plasma have been described, although in subjects with high altitude pulmonary oedema (see below) a raised ANP was consistently found.

7.8 Pathophysiological changes at altitude

7.8.1 Acute mountain sickness

Many people who ascend to altitudes above 2500 m, particularly when ascent is rapid, show a collection of symptoms referred to as acute mountain sickness or soroche. The symptoms, which include headache, nausea, vomiting, insomnia, somnolence, poor appetite, and muscle weakness, usually appear during the first 8–24 h at altitude, but occasionally may be delayed by up to 4 days. After abrupt exposure to moderate altitude (approximately 3000 m), approximately 30 per cent of individuals show symptoms but at an altitude of 4500 + m the incidence rises to 75 per cent. After 3–7 days the symptoms abate in the majority of sufferers. There seems to be no reliable characteristic to indicate whether or not an individual will develop acute mountain sickness, though in a given individual, the symptoms, if they appear, often appear with each altitude exposure.

The pathogenesis of acute mountain sickness is not clear, but the hypoxic conditions are considered to be the primary stimulus. In part, acute mountain sickness appears to be due to disturbances of body fluid distribution and volume regulation. On ascent to altitude there is increased secretion of ADH and adrenal corticoids (see previous section) which causes fluid retention. Coupled with the direct effects of hypoxia on the peripheral circulation, which lead to blood being shunted away from the periphery, there is accumulation of fluid in the lungs, splanchnic bed, and brain. As a result, these organs become mildly oedematous, which explains why many of the symptoms are related to dysfunction of these organs. Those individuals who do not develop an antidiuresis at altitude appear to remain well, again indicating that disturbed body fluid regulation seems to be a contributory factor to the development of acute mountain sickness.

Prevention of acute mountain sickness involves avoiding too rapid an ascent. A rate of ascent of 300 m per day at altitudes between 3000 and 4270 m and 150 m per day thereafter has been recommended, but pulmonary and cerebral oedema (see below) have still been reported even when these guidelines have been followed.

Acute mountain sickness can also be prevented by the use of drugs. Thus, both acetazolamide (a carbonic anhydrase inhibitor) and dexamethasone (a synthetic glucocorticoid) have been used successfully. It is believed that the former works by correcting the respiratory alkalosis which develops on first exposure to altitude, allowing the processes of acclimatization to occur more rapidly. The mode of action of dexamethasone appears to be via reduction in the cerebral oedema.

Once symptoms have appeared, the most successful remedy is to descend to a lower altitude or breathe oxygen (although even then symptoms do not disappear immediately, proving that acute mountain sickness is not due to hypoxia *per se*). Acetazolamide and dexamethasone have also been used successfully to treat patients with established symptoms.

7.8.2 High altitude pulmonary oedema

A further disease associated with ascent to altitude is pulmonary oedema, the first signs of which are marked dyspnoea and dry cough; when more severe, a foaming pink sputum is coughed up. Unless treated promptly, this disease may be fatal. It has been reported at altitudes of 2590 m, but its frequency increases with increasing altitude. Predisposing factors appear to be a rapid ascent, particularly in subjects who exercise in the cold and it is more frequent in younger than older subjects. The disease can occur not only in the unacclimatized visitor to altitude but also in HANs returning to altitude from a visit to sea-level for as little as 1 day.

The pathogenesis of this disease is not clearly understood, with susceptibility to the disease varying considerably between individuals. In part, it is caused by hypoxic vasoconstriction of pulmonary arteries and arterioles leading to a marked pulmonary hypertension. This, in turn, leads to increased filtration of fluid at the pulmonary capillaries. In addition, there appears to be an increase in pulmonary capillary permeability and inflammatory responses have been implicated.

The symptoms rapidly disappear with oxygen therapy or descent to a lower altitude, which remains the definitive treatment.

7.8.3 Chronic mountain sickness

Chronic mountain sickness or Monge's disease is a disease seen in the long-term resident at altitude and is therefore mostly seen in the HAN, particularly middle-aged men. There is no known treatment except to move the patient to a lower altitude.

Chronic mountain sickness is not a form of prolonged acute mountain sickness, rather its symptoms are associated with changes akin to the patient losing acclimatization. Thus, minute ventilation falls with a resultant fall in P_aO_2. This, in turn, stimulates erythropoiesis so that haematocrit rises to high values (as high as 80 per cent). Associated with this marked poly-cythaemia there is often a cyanosis. In addition, the pulmonary arterial hypertension, normally seen in the HAN, becomes exaggerated. Why these changes take place has not been elucidated but it is thought to be associated with the ageing process.

Further reading

Frisancho, A.R. (1975). Functional adaptation to high altitude. *Science*, **187**, 313–19.

Heath, D. and Williams, D.R. (1989). *High-altitude medicine and pathology*. Butterworths, London.

Lahiri, S. (1977). Physiological responses and adaptations to high altitude. In *Environmental physiology II*, International Review of Physiology, Vol. 15, (ed. D. Robertshaw), Chapter 7. University Park Press, Baltimore.

Monge, C. and Leon-Vearde, F. (1991). Physiological adaptation to high altitude: oxygen transport in mammals and birds. *Physiological Reviews*, **71**, 1135–72.

Ward, M.P., Milledge, J.S., and West, J.B. (1989). *High altitude medicine and physiology*. Chapman Hall Medical, London.

West, J.B. (1990). Tolerance to severe hypoxia: lessons from Mt Everest. *Acta Anaesthesiology Scandanavia*, **34**, Suppl. 94, 18–23.

8

Life underwater

8.1 Introduction

Although people do not live permanently underwater, some work long hours there, for example, the divers in North Sea oil operations and an ever increasing number of people are taking up diving for recreational purposes.

Like life at altitude, life underwater exposes people to a number of extreme conditions which are physiological stressors. These will be described briefly in a later section. However, a major change is a rise in ambient pressure. Such a hyperbaric environment can cause changes and raise problems due to the direct effects of pressure on the body. In addition, for normal breathing to continue, the diver must be supplied with a breathing mixture of gases at a pressure equal to ambient pressure. Breathing hyperbaric gases can also give rise to a number of problems. Collectively these problems are referred to as dysbarism.

This chapter will concentrate on the physiological changes and problems associated with life underwater. It should be noted, however, that many of these problems are also applicable to the 'compressed air' worker. That is, in the civil engineering industry it is sometimes necessary for construction workers to work in a sealed site in which the air pressure is elevated. For example, in the construction of a tunnel passing through highly porous strata, the workings are filled with compressed air to prevent penetration of water through the strata.

An understanding of the problems associated with work in a hyperbaric environment requires a knowledge of the physical principles associated with pressure.

8.2 Pressure—units of measurement and physical principles

The SI unit for pressure is the N/m^2 (equivalent to the Pa). However, when the partial pressures of inspired gases are considered, the mmHg (or its equivalent, the Torr) has been retained. In addition, since the N/m^2 is rather small, for convenience the bar has been adopted for expressing normal ambient pressures. (One bar is equivalent to 10^5 N/m^2, 750 mmHg and approximately 1 atmosphere.) However, in the diving industry, pressure is often described in terms of the depth in sea water, metres of sea water (msw).

The pressure at the bottom of a column of liquid can be calculated from:

$$\varrho g h$$

where ϱ is the density of the liquid, g is the acceleration of gravity, and h is the height of the column. Thus, in sea water (density 1.025), every 10 m of descent is associated with an increase in ambient pressure of approximately 1 bar. For example, assuming that normal atmospheric pressure is 1 bar, at a depth of 60 msw, the ambient pressure is 7 bar.

Since most of the body is composed of solids and liquids (mainly water) which are virtually incompressible, tissue pressures rise to the same extent as ambient pressure. As a result there is no danger that the body will be crushed (compressed) by the high ambient pressures found underwater. However, gases are compressible and follow Boyle's law (for a given mass of gas at constant temperature, its volume is inversely related to its pressure). Thus, during a breath-hold dive the **volume** of air in the lungs gradually decreases with increasing depth (increasing ambient pressure).

As the pressure of a given mass of gas is increased so its **density** (mass per unit volume) increases. In addition, in a mixture of gases, an increase in total gas pressure is associated with an increase in **partial pressures** of the constituent gases by the same proportion, according to Dalton's law. Finally, according to Henry's law, as the partial pressure of a gas is increased so the **amounts** of the gas dissolved in the body's liquids increase.

These physical principles give rise to a number of physiological as well as pathophysiological changes. For convenience, these changes will be considered in two sections:

(1) those due to the direct effects of pressure; and

(2) those due to breathing gases at an increased pressure.

8.3 The direct effects of increased pressure

8.3.1 Cardiovascular changes and the diving response

In the upright position with gravity acting through the longitudinal axis of the body, there is a hydrostatic pressure gradient down the body. Thus, blood pressure in the lower half of the body increases and results in the pooling of blood in these regions. However, when the body is surrounded by water there is an equal **external** hydrostatic pressure gradient down the body. This opposes the **internal** hydrostatic pressure gradient. As a result, when a person is immersed in water approximately 500 ml of blood moves from the lower half of the body to the thoracic regions. (This is the same shift of blood volume which occurs when a person rapidly moves from the upright to supine position.) The increase in central blood volume raises right atrial pressure and, consequently, stroke volume and cardiac output increase. The resulting increases in pulmonary blood flow and blood volume lead to an increased pulmonary diffusing capacity and, possibly also, an improved ventilation/perfusion ratio.

The increased central blood volume also leads, via stretch of atrial receptors, to a decrease in the release of vasopressin (ADH) and increased secretion of atrial natriuretic hormone. As a result, a diuresis develops (which explains why shortly after getting into the local public swimming baths, one often finds it necessary to get out again to micturate—although some people seem to make alternative arrangements!).

On first immersion in water, particularly when it is colder than 15°C, the heart rate falls (sometimes quite dramatically), breathing ceases, and selective vasoconstriction occurs, particularly in the skin. These changes are termed the 'diving response'. The response is caused by stimulation of cutaneous receptors on the face by cold water rather than a direct effect of pressure. It is greatly developed in diving mammals such as the seal and whale. Its adaptive role in these species is that it helps conserve oxygen by decreasing the work load of the heart and decreasing blood flow to most of the systemic circulation except for the strongest autoregulators, namely, the heart and brain. Thus, they are able to stay underwater for long periods.

8.3.2 Mechanics of breathing

The ambient pressure gradient down the thorax when a person is upright in water exaggerates the normal gradient in intrapleural pressure from the apex to the base of the lungs. In addition, if a person stands up to their neck in water (head-out immersion), such that alveolar pressure is approximately equal to normal atmospheric pressure, the increased pressure outside the chest opposes the outward elastic record of the chest wall. As a result function residual capacity is reduced, mostly at the expense of the expiratory reserve volume. In addition, with head-out immersion, the increased extra-thoracic pressure increases the work of breathing by approximately 60 per cent. These changes do not occur when an individual is supplied with air at a pressure equal to the ambient pressure at the level of the chest since, under these conditions, transthoracic pressures are normal. However, as will be seen in a later section, the breathing of hyperbaric gases can markedly alter the work of breathing.

8.3.3 Barotrauma

In addition to the physiological changes described above, a hyperbaric environment can directly lead to pathological changes and damage. These are referred to as barotrauma.

As mentioned above, gases in the body try to obey Boyle's law when exposed to changed ambient pressures. Gases in body cavities which are bounded by flexible membranes (for example, in the lungs and gastro-intestinal tract) are free to obey this law. Thus, during a breath-hold dive, as a person goes deeper the volume of air in the lungs decreases. Provided that the volume of lung gases are not compressed beyond residual volume, there is no problem. However, diving beyond that point causes a negative intra-alveolar pressure to develop, leading to 'lung squeeze'—pulmonary congestion, oedema, and haemorrhage.

During ascent from a breath-hold dive, the gases in the lung re-expand to their original volume causing no problem. By contrast, when a diver has been provided with compressed air (or some other gas mixture) during diving in order to continue normal breathing, pulmonary barotrauma can occur during ascent. Provided that the diver continues normal breathing during ascent, no problem occurs. However, if the diver fails to exhale during an ascent or gas is trapped in an area of the lung due to some pathology, such as a cyst or bulla, then the expanding gases may exceed the normal capacity of the lungs, leading to alveolar rupture. Such 'burst lung' usually occurs when intra-alveolar pressure exceeds ambient pressure by approximately 80 mmHg (11 kPa); this may occur from a dive to only 2 m.

Once the alveoli have ruptured the gas may escape to various sites. It may track to the hilum of the lungs via the perivascular sheaths and, thence, pass into the mediastinum. Pneumothorax may also result from gas escaping into the pleural cavity. Alternatively or additionally, gas may escape into the pulmonary circulation whence it reaches the systemic circulation via the left heart. Owing to the buoyancy of gases, such gas will normally pass upwards via the carotid arteries to the cerebral circulation causing cerebral arterial gas embolism. In this case, stroke-like symptoms appear and often consciousness is rapidly lost. This is a medical emergency and is treated by recompression to a pressure of 6 bar. Without the complications of cerebral gas embolism, the signs of pulmonary barotrauma are usually chest pain, cough, and, more rarely, dyspnoea.

Like gases in the lungs, gases in the intestinal tract will be compressed during a dive and re-expand again during surfacing. Usually no problems arise, although if extra gas is produced in the intestinal tract during the dive the expansion of this during surfacing may give rise to mild abdominal discomfort and flatulence (so stay away from a diver who has had baked beans for breakfast!).

There are some gas-containing cavities in the body which are not free to undergo any change in volume because they are bounded by rigid structures, for example, in the middle ear and paranasal sinuses. If the pressure of the gas in such a cavity cannot equilibrate with ambient pressure during a descent the resulting transmural pressure gives rise to the risk of damage to the suspending structures. A more immediate problem, however, is the effect on the vasculature in the mucosal lining of the cavity. The large transmural pressure across the vasculature will lead to exudation of fluid and, if sufficiently great, may even lead to rupture of capillaries.

Normally barotrauma of the middle ear is prevented by equilibrating the pressure in the middle ear with ambient pressure. Such equilibration normally occurs automatically via the Eustachian tube but can be aided by yawning or performing the Frenzel or Valsalva manoeuvres ('popping the ears'). However, if the entrance to the Eustachian tube is blocked or inflamed, for example, by an upper respiratory infection, equilibration may become impossible and damage may occur. As a descent continues, a significant pressure gradient will develop across the tympanic membrane causing it to bulge inward, resulting in pain. In addition, there may be haemorrhage of the tympanic membrane or, with a sufficient pressure gradient, it may perforate. This may take place with a pressure gradient of as little as 100 mmHg (13 kPa), which can occur at a depth of only 3 msw.

A much more serious, but fortunately rare, form of otic barotrauma is associated with rupture of the oval or round window. This can occur with over-vigorous attempts to 'pop' the ears during descent. Such damage leads to sudden onset of vertigo, tinnitus, and deafness on the affected side.

As with the middle ear, if the channels connecting the paranasal sinuses to the nasopharynx are blocked, as in sinusitis, equalization of pressure between the sinuses and the nasal passages cannot occur, leading to transudation and haemorrhage of the lining of the sinuses accompanied by exquisite pain. The frontal and maxillary sinuses are most commonly affected.

Barotrauma can develop in any air-filled cavity that does not equilibrate with ambient pressure. For example, if the diver wears air-tight goggles which are restricted to the eyes, with descent there is likely to be conjunctival damage. Further, when a diving helmet is used, another danger is that of classical 'diver's squeeze'. This occurs when the air supply to the helmet becomes inadequate, perhaps as a result of some mechanical failure in a pump. As the air pressure in the helmet falls relative to ambient pressure, the external water pressure tends to force the whole of the diver into it.

8.3.4 High pressure neurological syndrome (HPNS)

Although the body solids and liquids can be considered virtually incompressible, they are not absolutely so. In particular, lipids are more compressible than water. Thus, at very high pressures, lipids may be compressed slightly. Compression of lipids in the cell membranes of neurones, with resulting changes in permeability and transport properties, is thought to be responsible for the symptoms referred to as high pressure neurological syndrome. These symptoms include tremor, decreased manual dexterity, dizziness, loss of attentiveness, and nausea. Such symptoms are normally seen at pressures of over 21 bar (200 msw) and are more frequent and severe with increasing pressure and when the rate of descent is rapid. The symptoms may be lessened by the addition of a small amount of nitrogen to the helium–oxygen mixtures (see later) which are usually breathed at these extreme depths.

8.4 The effects of breathing hyperbaric gases

When air is breathed via a snorkel, a dive below 0.5 m is unsafe. This is because the increase in ambient pressure which occurs with increasing depth diminishes the volume of air in the lungs, according to Boyle's law. To prevent the diminution in lung volume, the inspiratory muscles must exert a greater pressure (equal to the increase in ambient pressure). The greatest pressure that can be generated by the inspiratory muscles is approximately 90 mmHg (12 kPa); when ambient pressure exceeds this value (at a depth of 1.2 m), inspiration of air from the surface is impossible. In practice the maximum safe depth for breathing air from the surface is less than 1 m for two reasons. Firstly, when alveolar pressure is much less than ambient pressure 'lung squeeze' may occur and, secondly, a snorkel greater than 0.5 m in length increases deadspace to such an extent that alveolar ventilation will become inadequate.

In dives deeper than 0.5 m, therefore, the diver must be supplied with a breathing mixture at a pressure equal to ambient pressure. In recreational SCUBA diving, the diver inspires from a cylinder of compressed air (21 per cent O_2, 79 per cent N_2). As the diver goes deeper, a demand valve ensures that air is provided at a pressure to match ambient pressure. In the deep sea diver, involved in work underwater for several hours, a breathing mixture is fed to the diver from the surface via a hose, the pressure of the breathing mixture again being maintained the same as the ambient pressure. However, breathing gases under pressure is not without its problems because, with increasing pressure:

(1) the density of gases increases;

(2) the partial pressure of the inspired gases increases.

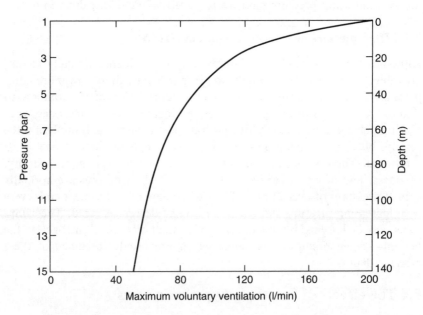

Fig. 8.1. Changes in maximum voluntary ventilation with increasing pressure and depth.

Each of these can produce further problems which may limit the depth of a dive.

8.4.1 The effects of increased air density

As the density of inspired gases increases so, for a given tidal volume, a greater mass of gases is moved. This increases the inspiratory effort and so the work of breathing. Thus, maximal voluntary ventilation (MVV) decreases with increasing depth, the decrement being approximately proportional to the reciprocal of the square root of the density (Fig. 8.1).

Breathing air of increased density increases the work of breathing in another way; as the density of air rises so the likelihood of turbulent flow increases (cf. Reynolds number). Turbulent flow increases airway resistance. This, together with an increased external resistance of the breathing apparatus, increases the work of breathing. Finally, air of increased density slows intra-alveolar diffusion of gases.

All in all, these effects lead to a reduced maximum aerobic capacity ($\dot{V}O_2$max), the limitation being set by ventilatory rather than cardiovascular factors (the latter are normally limiting at sea-level).

The reduction in ventilatory performance can be attenuated by replacing the nitrogen in inspired air by helium, which is less dense (see later).

8.4.2 The effects of increased partial pressure of gases

8.4.2.1 *Nitrogen narcosis*

When compressed air is used to sustain breathing during diving, the diver runs the risk of nitrogen narcosis which develops progressively as the partial pressure of nitrogen increases. In most individuals, initial symptoms occur at a depth of 30 msw (4 bar), but some divers show signs at as little as 10 msw. These symptoms, which have been termed 'raptures of the deep', resemble alcohol intoxication: a feeling of euphoria, irrational behaviour, reduced dexterity, and mental agility. Down to a depth of 50 msw (6 bar) the impairment is usually mild with perhaps some loss of concentration and decrease in neuromuscular co-ordination. Beyond 50 msw, however, the symptoms become more marked and, at depths beyond 90 msw, most divers approach unconsciousness. For this reason, legislation in most countries limits commercial diving using compressed air to a depth of 50 m.

How nitrogen produces narcosis is not completely understood but is thought to be similar to that of anaesthetic gases. That is, being soluble in lipids, nitrogen causes a small but significant change in membrane volume. This leads to modulation of ion channels and consequent disruption of the excitability of axons and impairment of synaptic transmission. It is interesting to note that HPNS (see earlier) is also thought to be caused by a change (decrease) in cell volume, suggesting that there is a 'critical volume' for normal cell membrane function.

8.4.2.2 *Oxygen toxicity*

It might be thought that nitrogen narcosis could be avoided and dives safely extended beyond a depth of 50 msw, by breathing pure oxygen. Unfortunately this is not the case because oxygen becomes toxic at increased partial pressures. In the context of diving, toxicity at two sites needs to be considered: the lungs and the central nervous system.

When inspired PO_2 rises above 1350 mmHg (1.8 bar), which occurs at a depth of only 8 msw when pure oxygen is being breathed, oxygen is toxic to the nervous system and can rapidly cause epileptiform convulsions. Sometimes these convulsions are preceded by vertigo, nausea, paraesthesia of the arms or legs, and twitching of muscles round the eyes or mouth. The latent period before the development of convulsions decreases with increasing inspired PO_2 and with physical exertion.

The mechanism by which oxygen is toxic to the CNS is not fully understood but is thought to be due to oxidation of sulphydryl groups in some enzymes and in membrane proteins. This leads to disruption of function and hyperexcitability of neurones.

When breathing pure oxygen, diving is obviously limited to a depth of 8 msw. In practice only the military use pure oxygen as an inspired gas. This is used in a closed-circuit, rebreathing apparatus to prevent tell-tale bubbles at the surface during clandestine operations!

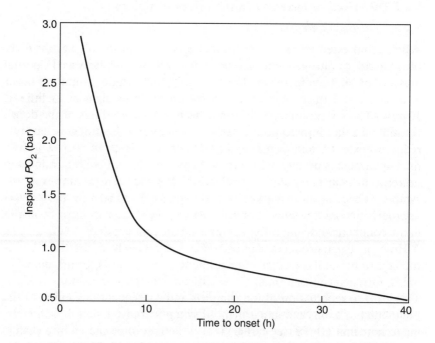

Fig. 8.2. Time to onset of symptoms of pulmonary oxygen toxicity at different inspired PO_2s.

When breathed over a long period, even more modest PO_2s can be toxic to the lungs. The initial symptom of pulmonary oxygen toxicity is coughing but this worsens to dyspnoea and eventually pulmonary oedema and intra-alveolar haemorrhage, which may be fatal. The symptoms are caused by progressive destruction of alveolar endothelial and epithelial cells. Pulmonary toxicity can develop when inspired PO_2 is as little as 375 mmHg (0.5 bar), such as that found at a depth of 16 msw if compressed air is breathed. However, at such a PO_2, symptoms only appear after more than 30 h. With increasing PO_2s, the latency decreases so that symptoms occur after 5 h when inspired PO_2 is 1500 mmHg (2 bar) (Fig. 8.2).

8.4.2.3 *Use of helium–oxygen mixtures (heliox)*

Below a depth of 50 msw, breathing compressed air is dangerous because of the likelihood of nitrogen narcosis (see earlier). Replacement of nitrogen by oxygen is not a solution because of oxygen's toxicity. Therefore, in dives below 50 msw, commercial divers breath a helium–oxygen mixture. Helium is used since it has only approximately one-eighth the narcotic effects of nitrogen, so that much higher partial pressures can be withstood. The ratio of helium to oxygen in the heliox mixture is adjusted so that inspired PO_2 does not exceed approximately 300 mmHg (0.4 bar). Thus, for example, at a depth of 100 msw (11 bar) the percentage oxygen in the heliox mixture is only approximately 4.4 per cent; at a depth of 300 msw (31 bar) a mere 1.26 per cent oxygen is used.

Besides its very small narcotic potential, there are other advantages in the use of helium rather than nitrogen as the diluent gas. First, helium has only one-seventh the density of nitrogen so that the work of breathing is reduced (see earlier). Second, the solubility of helium is only approximately 40 per cent that of nitrogen. Together with the decreased density and, therefore, diffusibility, this decreased solubility reduces the likelihood of decompression sickness developing (see next section). However, because of its low density, breathing helium elevates the pitch of the voice (giving it a 'Donald Duck' sound) which makes verbal communication difficult, if perhaps amusing! Helium also has high thermal conductivity which leads to considerably increased respiratory heat losses.

8.4.3 Decompression sickness

8.4.3.1 *Gas uptake and elimination*

When gases are breathed under pressure, more of the gases dissolve in the body fluids, in accordance with Dalton's Law. Thus, for example, when breathing air at sea-level the body contains approximately 1 l of nitrogen in solution of the body's water, but this increases by a further litre for every 10 m descent (every 1 bar increase in pressure) when compressed air is breathed. However, the new equilibrium is not attained immediately. This is because blood volume is only 8 per cent of total body volume and so considerable time is taken for enough nitrogen to be transported from the lungs to the tissues for them to reach equilibrium at the new partial pressure of nitrogen. As well as being time- and pressure-dependent, the rate and quantity of gas taken up by any particular tissue also depends upon the rate of perfusion and the solubility coefficient of the tissue. Thus, for example, well perfused tissues, such as the brain, take up nitrogen and reach equilibrium quickly, whereas adipose tissue, which has a lower perfusion, reaches equilibrium much more slowly. The time taken for all the tissues to reach equilibrium is theoretically a constant and usually considered to be 6–8 h, although a substantial proportion of the extra gas uptake will have occurred before this time. Diving in which the tissues reach this equilibrium is referred to as saturation diving. (Note that saturation diving does not imply saturation in its usual context, that is, that no more gas can be taken up; rather it implies that the tissues have reached equilibrium with the new alveolar gas pressure).

The problem for the diver is not associated with the uptake of extra gases, rather it is to eliminate them when decompression takes place on ascent. As the diver ascends and inspired gas pressures fall, a partial pressure gradient for gases develops between tissues and alveoli. Thus, the extra gas in the body fluids taken up during compression will diffuse from the tissues into the blood and be eliminated at the lungs. However, in the same way that the uptake of gases during compression is not immediate, so too during decompression there is a maximal rate at which the gases can be eliminated. Therefore, if the quantity of gases dissolved in the tissues is large and the rate of ascent is rapid, so that ambient and tissue pressure fall rapidly, the tissues will become supersaturated with gases causing the gases to come out of solution and form bubbles (just as when a bottle of champagne is opened). It is the appearance of these bubbles which cause decompression sickness (often also referred to as 'the bends', though in fact 'the bends' are only one manifestation of decompression sickness). Of particular importance is the appearance of bubbles of inert gas which cannot be utilized by the tissues, particularly nitrogen when compressed air has been breathed. If oxygen bubbles form, these can be used locally in tissue metabolism and carbon dioxide bubbles do not form since there is little of this gas in inspired air.

8.4.3.2 *Development and symptoms of decompression sickness*

While the underlying cause of decompression sickness is the formation of inert gas bubbles, how these bubbles then cause the various symptoms of decompression sickness is still uncertain. Thus, when bubble formation has been measured in divers using Doppler techniques, formation of bubbles has not always been associated with any overt symptoms. Furthermore, the same diver can undergo the same dive with the same rate of decompression on different days and suffer overt symptoms on one day but not on another (although symptoms will always occur if the rate of ascent is too rapid). Overt symptoms may be related to whether or not the bubbles reach some critical size.

In addition to a rapid ascent, other factors which predispose to decompression sickness are obesity, poor physical condition, age, and exertion. Professional divers who undergo frequent decompression appear less likely to complain of symptoms but this may simply be an habituation (a raised threshold) to pain.

Various hypotheses have been advanced, which alone or in combination, may explain why bubbles cause decompression sickness.

1. Direct mechanical effects of extracellular gas bubbles, distorting tissues, and/or blocking capillaries.
2. Cellular damage due to intracellular gases.
3. Changes in the vascular endothelium and aggregation of intravascular fat, imposed by intravascular bubbles.
4. A host of changes induced in blood by the gas–liquid interface between the surface of a bubble and blood. This can involve, for example, activation of blood platelets, the complement system, and kinins.

The onset of signs and symptoms of decompression sickness may not occur until 36 h after decompression but 90 per cent appear within 6 h. One of the most common symptoms is pain in the joints of the extremities due to the formation of bubbles in the tendons and ligaments. The diver refers to these symptoms as 'bends' when the pain is severe or 'niggles' when it is mild. In divers the pain is usually felt in the shoulder or elbow joints whereas in the compressed air worker it is more usual in the knee joint.

Larger intravascular bubbles usually get trapped in the pulmonary vascular bed. Here they can block pulmonary capillaries giving rise to severe dyspnoea and cough, referred to by the diver as 'chokes'.

A serious form of decompression sickness is when bubbles form in the spinal cord or when intravascular bubbles block the circulation to the cord. The resulting degeneration of nerve fibres can cause any combination of motor or sensory deficits. When marked, this can lead to permanent paralysis which is often in the lower half of the body. More rarely, there may be vertigo, referred to by divers as 'staggers', due to bubble formation in the vestibular apparatus.

A further long-term health problem associated with decompression sickness is avascular necrosis of bone. This is thought to be the result of bubbles blocking the end arteries of bone as a result of which the bone dies. Usually the lesion is in the head, neck, or shaft of long bones, particular the upper humerus, upper and lower femur, and upper tibia. In a small number of cases the bone under the articular surface may be affected, which may lead to serious arthritic problems in the shoulder and hip joints.

8.4.3.3 *Avoidance of decompression sickness*

The avoidance of decompression sickness depends upon selecting a rate of ascent that precludes significant bubble formation. In practice divers use 'Decompression Tables'. Most of these are derived from early observations made in 1908 by Haldane based partly on experimental observations in animals and partly on calculations of how nitrogen is washed out of the body. Haldane suggested that significant bubble formation would not occur if total tissue gas pressure did not exceed twice the ambient pressure. Thus, Decompression Tables requires an ascent being made in several stages, with 'stops' at depths where the ambient pressure is half that at the depth of the previous stop. At each stop sufficient time is allowed for the inert gases to be eliminated from the body until equilibrium is again attained. The number of stops and the time at each stop (which are more rigorous than proposed by Haldane) are determined by the depth to which the diver has been and how long he has been there. For example, a dive to 20 msw for 2 h requires two stops and decompression takes in total approximately 50 min, whereas a dive to 50 msw for only 45 min requires five stops and a total 85 min decompression. With more extreme depths the decompression times are several hours, even with short dives. For this reason, saturation diving is increasingly used for dives below 50 msw. That is, the diver is kept under pressure for longer periods by transferring to a chamber maintained at the same ambient pressure as the water he emerged from. In North Sea operations a diver may be maintained under pressure for as long as 4 weeks. The subsequent decompression times are very long, taking approximately 4 days for saturation diving at 100 msw and 10 days for diving at 300 msw.

The risk of decompression sickness is reduced if heliox is breathed during the dive (essential in dives below 50 msw to avoid nitrogen narcosis). Helium is approximately 40 per cent as soluble as nitrogen so that less dissolves in the tissues. In addition, since helium has one-seventh of the molecular weight of nitrogen, it diffuses two and a half times more rapidly through the tissues and therefore it can be eliminated more rapidly during decompression.

A diver must also avoid flying in an aircraft for some time after diving. This is because the ambient pressure in an aircraft is less than normal atmospheric pressure at sea-level (see Chapter 7) and the further decrease in ambient pressure may cause bubble formation. Indeed, decompression sickness is sometimes observed in military aviators since the cockpit pressure in military aircraft is allowed to fall lower than that in civil aircraft.

8.5 Other problems associated with diving

The underwater environment presents other challenges to those who work there. The density of water increases the effort required for any movement. Due to the buoyancy of the body in water, the diver is, in effect, weightless whilst underwater. (It is for this reason that astronauts train underwater, see Chapter 9.) This weightlessness makes it difficult to use tools which produce torque. Visibility under water is impaired in several ways. First, the face mask will restrict the field of vision. Second, the change in refractive index between water and the glass of a face mask distorts perception of size and distance. Finally, below a depth of 30 msw only the blue–green bands of the spectrum of daylight penetrate and scattering of light and visibility will be hindered further by pollutants in the water. Hearing is also impaired because, although sound travels four times faster in water than in air, sound attenuation is much greater so that the diver hears little other than the sound of his own breathing. This also produces disorientation.

A further major physiological problem to be overcome is cold. The water surrounding the diver conducts heat away from the body surface. Some protection can be afforded by the use of a wet suit but the thermal insulation provided by this decreases with increasing depth since the increased pressure compresses the suit. When heliox is breathed, heat loss is exaggerated because of the increased respiratory heat loss due to helium's high thermal conductivity and capacity. Thus, with deep sea diving (sea temperature falls with increasing depth) it is often necessary to give the diver his own central heating system by providing him with an electrically heated suit or piping hot water through the diving suit. In addition, it may be necessary to heat the breathing mixture to decrease the respiratory losses.

It is no wonder that the job done by commercial divers is one which many of us do not envy.

Further reading

Bennett, P.B. and Elliott, D.H. (ed.) (1983). *The physiology and medicine of diving*. 3rd edn, Balliere Tindall, London.

Calder, I.M. (1986). Dysbarism. A review. *Forensic Science International*, **30**, 237–66.

Elliott, D.H. (1981). Underwater physiology. In *The Principles and Practice of Human Physiology*. (ed. O.G. Edholm and J.S. Weiner), Ch. 6. Academic Press, London.

Smith, E.B. (1986). Priestley lecture 1986. On the science of deep-sea diving—observations on the respiration of different kinds of air. *Undersea Biomedical Research*, **14**, 347–69.

Strauss, R.H. (1979). Diving medicine. *American Review of Respiratory Disorders*, **119**, 1001–23.

9

Acceleration forces

9.1 Changing G-forces

When a person stands up quickly from a lying position, they are in danger of fainting due to an inadequate supply of blood to the brain. The reason for this is that the Earth's gravitational field causes pooling of blood in the legs and, hence, a decrease in venous return. The apparatus for studying these changes—the tilt table—and the corrective reflexes that come into operation—the baroreceptor reflexes—are described in standard textbooks of physiology. Here we shall consider the cause of these changes, how the body responds to them, and how they can be combated when the body is subjected to a force other than the 1-G force always acting towards the centre of the Earth.

Such changes in G-forces arise when the individual is being accelerated or retarded (deaccelerated). From one of Newton's Laws of Motion, any movement, for example, ascent in a lift or the 'spring' in a person's gait, causes a force to be exerted upon the body. These forces are transient and small. The development of fast transport has increased them. In normal journeys by car, the forces due to acceleration, braking, and cornering can last for several seconds but are rarely greater than 1-G (that is, equal to the force exerted by gravity) and they act sideways and backwards or forwards rather than upwards or downwards. Similar forces are experienced in commercial flights. For test pilots and those involved in aerial displays or combat, transient forces up to 8-G are not uncommon and can act for several seconds. Generally these forces act in a headwards direction—as when a plane is turning and the head of the pilot is tilting towards the centre of rotation—but they can act in the opposite direction—as when the pilot is flying 'upside-down' or circling with his head pointing away from the centre of rotation. At fairgrounds, some people seem to enjoy experiencing increased G-forces! Here the forces are rarely more than 2- or 3-G but they can be experienced for minutes at a time and act in all directions. The advent of rocket travel requires headwards acceleration forces to be experienced for several minutes during the launch and during re-entry into the Earth's atmosphere after a flight.

Decreased G-forces can also be experienced, for example, at the start of descents during a fairground ride or from the crest of a wave when sailing. A special case exists when the body is falling freely, that is, when the condition of zero-G or 'weightlessness' is experienced. This occurs in satellites orbiting the Earth and can exist for weeks or more. Like cosmonauts, bed-ridden patients are also not subjected to the normal pooling of blood in dependent limbs. In both cases, it is important to establish if this causes any longer term physiological changes. Not only is this relevant to patient care but it might indicate whether or not it would be possible for interplanetary travel, which would require living in a zero-G environment for months or even years.

In considering the changes in blood flow that accompany these changes in G-forces, it is important to remember that in any column of fluid there is a difference in pressure, *P*, between two points given by the equation:

$$P = h \varrho G$$

where *P* can be conveniently expressed as cm H_2O, *h* is the distance (cm) measured in the direction of the acceleration force, ϱ is the density of the fluid (g/cm^3), and *G* is the acceleration force acting upon the column (expressed as a multiple of the normal gravitational force).

It is clear from this equation that the pressure gradient varies in size and direction in accordance with the acceleration forces acting upon the body and the orientation of the body with respect to the direction of acceleration. Not only does this mean the gradient will disappear in the weightless condition but also it indicates ways in which the effects of the acceleration forces can be reduced. Both of these areas will be considered later.

9.2 Increased G-forces

9.2.1 Means of study

The method that has been used to study increased G-forces is to sit the subject in a huge centrifuge (Fig. 9.1). With this apparatus, the force exerted can be determined from the radius of the turning circle and the speed of rotation. Even though the Earth's gravitational force continues to act vertically, the direction in which the imposed centripetal force acts depends upon the subject's posture. Much work has been concerned with the effects of headwards acceleration, in which the subject's head tilts towards the centre of rotation of the centrifuge.

9.2.2 The central nervous system

If a subject is suddenly accelerated in a headwards direction with a force of approximately 4-G, peripheral vision is impaired within a few seconds and perception of colour and detail by the fovea deteriorates. These symptoms are generally called 'grey-out'. With a higher acceleration (4.5 to 5-G), vision, but not consciousness, is lost (black-out); above 5-G, unconsciousness results. These changes are caused by inadequate blood flow to the eyes and brain. The immediate effect of the headwards acceleration is to cause a fall in the intraluminal pressure since the deficit below aortic pressure $h \varrho G$, will be increased by the raised value of G. Other factors are important also. The fact that the arteries in the eye radiate outwards from the optic nerve means that the vessels supplying the retinal periphery are longer. Length is inevitably associated with resistance, as a result of which intraluminal pressures will tend to be lower and so the vessels will always be more susceptible to collapse. Finally, the position is worsened by the intraocular fluid whose pressure (approximately 20 cm H_2O) decreases the transmural

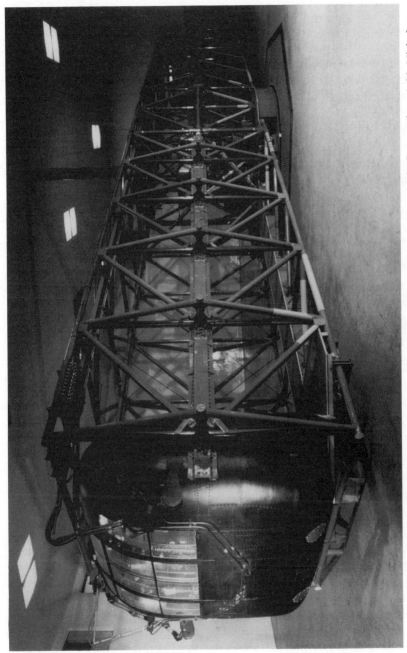

Fig. 9.1. RAF Institute of Aviation Medicine, human centrifuge. By kind permission of Air Commodore A.N. Nicholson, RAF, O.B.E.

pressure gradient. The combination of all these factors means that the pressure across the vessel walls falls to below the critical closing pressure. It is to be noted that, since the venous pressure falls by an amount similar to that in the arteries, the change in arteriovenous pressure differences is small. In other words, it is the fall in intraluminal pressure and rise in vessel resistance, not a fall in perfusion pressure, that causes the retinal blood supply to fail.

Brain function in general is less susceptible than vision to the effects of acceleration (for example, consciousness is maintained during 'black-out'). This is because the perfusion of the brain vascular bed is better preserved than that to the eyes for a number of reasons.

1. The brain is surrounded by an indistensible skull and its centre is filled with fluid (the cerebrospinal fluid). The hydrostatic pressure in this fluid changes by an amount equal to that in the blood vessels. Therefore, because pressures in the brain interstitial fluid reflect cerebrospinal fluid pressure much more closely than intravascular pressure, there is little change in transmural pressure and, as a consequence, vessel calibre. (The eyes, of course, are outside the skull, and so are not protected by this mechanism.)

2. In the brain as in the eye, the arteriovenous difference in pressure is preserved because the venous pressure falls as much as the arterial pressure. However, blood flow drops dramatically when forces in excess of 5-G are experienced (see above). This is probably because, with this amount of acceleration, the pressure produced by the heart has largely been dissipated by the time the base of the skull has been reached, so the vessels collapse.

3. If brain perfusion does decrease, autoregulation of vascular tone occurs (initiated by local gas tension and metabolite changes) and is very marked.

Therefore, provided that the vessels do not collapse, blood flow to the brain is maintained surprisingly well, though deterioration in mental performance before unconsciousness occurs has been measured in some studies. If the blood vessels do collapse, then unconsciousness occurs very rapidly.

After approximately 5–10 s of acceleration, blood flow to the brain and eyes begins to recover as a result of baroreceptor reflexes. These are also important when acceleration forces are increased only slowly, when they enable cerebral and retinal blood flow to be maintained during forces reaching 6-G. The major stimuli to reflex activity are changes in blood pressure monitored by the carotid sinuses. The baroreceptors of the aortic arch are likely to be far less effective since they are not positioned above the heart. Indeed, some have suggested that, since they are effectively *below* the heart and so will monitor a raised blood pressure, they will act to reduce the size of the reflex response.

9.2.3 The cardiovascular and respiratory systems

An immediate consequence of headwards acceleration is a decrease in cardiac output. Acceleration causes the internal organs of the body to move away from the head; this reduces intrathoracic pressure. Even though the pulse pressure developed during cardiac systole remains the same, it is taking place against a reduction in intrathoracic pressure and so there is a net fall in driving force to areas outside the thorax. Other early changes include an increased pooling of blood in the dependent parts of the body, with decreased venous return as a consequence. Both changes contribute to the fall in blood pressure in the carotid sinus and the baroreceptor reflex that this induces.

Acceleration also affects breathing movements and respiratory gas exchange. With headwards acceleration, the movement of internal organs facilitates inspiration, by pulling down the diaphragm, but hinders expiration. Not surprisingly tidal volume tends to encroach upon the inspiratory reserve. Acceleration away from the head produces the opposite effects, inspiration now becoming more difficult.

The lung shows gradients of blood perfusion and alveolar ventilation; both increase from its apex to its base in a normal 1-G environment. These gradients of perfusion and ventilation are both produced by factors which are affected by acceleration forces. Acceleration in a headwards direction accentuates the gradients whereas accleration in the opposite direction can reverse them. During headwards acceleration, the apical alveoli will be almost fully distended throughout the respiratory cycle but receive very little ventilation and even zero perfusion; since their perfusion will approach zero, their ventilation/perfusion ratio will be abnormally high. By contrast, the basal parts of the lung receive large amounts of blood (so much so that there is even the possibility of pulmonary oedema), but ventilation, even though it rises, does not do so proportionally and a lowered ventilation/perfusion ratio is the result. As a result of these changes, the apex and base of the lung function poorly with respect to gas exchange. Alveolar deadspace at the apex and venous shunts at the base cause ventilatory and cardiac work to be wasted and hypoxaemia and even ischaemia develop.

9.2.4 Countermeasures

The major problems with acceleration are caused by the redistribution of blood flow in accord with pressure changes given by the term $h\varrho G$. If it is possible for a person to accelerate 'forwards' rather than headwards, pressure gradients will be lessened because the thickness of the body is less than its height. In practice this requires the cosmonaut or pilot to be in a supine rather than a sitting position. Obviously, some degree of compromise might be required if tasks have to be performed but a greater tolerance to G-forces has been found when the body is positioned in this way.

Preventing the fall in cardiac output must be another aim. This can be achieved in several ways. First, transient Valsalva manoeuvres (that is, forced expiration against a closed glottis) and shouting both raise intra-thoracic pressure, as does positive pressure breathing. These methods are all effective in increasing cardiac output for a few beats and this might be sufficient. But if the countermeasure is needed for more than a few seconds, then it is necessary to increase venous return. This can be achieved by tensing the leg and thigh muscles, though this is not possible when the legs are required for other purposes, such as piloting a helicopter. An artificial aid that has been developed to combat the fall in venous return for extended periods of time is the 'antigravity suit'. It is based upon the principle that immersing a person in water counters the gravitational effects already described by producing an equal hydrostatic gradient outside the body. This would leave unchanged the transmural pressure across the veins and, there-fore, the volume of blood they hold. Recent designs have been air-filled rather than water-filled and have tended not to encase the lower body com-pletely. Antigravity suits are believed to work not only because they prevent venous pooling but also because they limit the descent of the diaphragm. This keeps the heart nearer to the head, so decreasing the amount of pres-sure required to drive blood up to the brain.

Recent work has shown that combinations of these different counter-measures are most effective.

A further countermeasure can be taken to reduce visual disturbances. Goggles can be worn that enable the extraocular pressure (and, hence, the pressure surrounding the retinal vessels) to be changed. Decreases in extra-ocular pressure act to promote retinal blood flow and combat high G-forces in the headwards direction, by maintaining the transmural pressure gradient in retinal vessels. Conversely, if the pilot is flying upside down so that intra-luminal and transmural pressure gradients are increased, raised pressure in the goggles maintains the transmural pressure gradient and retinal vessel resistance at normal values.

9.3 Physiological effects of weightlessness

If we are to explore the solar system, we shall have to endure weightlessness for months or even years. Can we adjust to such periods of zero-G and, if so, what happens when we return to live again in a gravitational field? Such questions might seem rather esoteric but a similar problem exists for patients who are bedridden for extended periods of time. Even though they are still subject to gravity, it no longer acts along the length of their bodies but rather across the width. What changes occur in these patients and what happens when they have recovered enough to stand and walk again?

9.3.1 Means of study

Before the first manned space flight it was necessary to have some idea of how cosmonauts would react to weightlessness over a period of at least a few days. Earth-bound investigators used constant bed-rest and water-immersion techniques to mimic the effects of weightlessness. When using a complete bed-rest regimen, it is better to have the volunteers tilted at 6° to the horizontal with their head down, rather than in a horizontal posture. This is because in this position the carotid sinuses are level with the aortic valve, rather than slightly above it. This reduces the pressure difference, $h\varrho G$, to zero and so mimics the effects of zero-gravity more accurately. Studies lasting up to 190 days have been performed. A major difficulty with this method is in deciding what changes in posture should be allowed for meals and toilet and for carrying out tasks that might be required in an orbiting satellite. Patients who have been immobilized during recovery from ligament operations also provide useful information but patients recovering from bone fractures or coma are less useful because of the interpretive difficulties that might arise. The comatose patient can hardly be regarded as normal and there would be considerable doubts as to how 'normal' were bone changes (see below) in somebody recovering from a fracture.

Water-immersion studies, the rationale for which is identical to that for the 'antigravity suit' already discussed, suffer from different problems. Thus, the temperature of the water affects considerably the subjects' comfort and ability to sweat; subjects have to be separated from the water by an impervious sheet to prevent damage to the skin and movement is difficult because of the viscosity of the water.

In spite of these problems, results from these types of study are similar to those obtained so far in the prolonged space flights (up to 1 year) of the Soyuz, Salyut, Skylab, Spacelab, and Mir programmes. For this reason, the results from all techniques are assumed to be identical unless it is stated otherwise.

9.3.2 Body fluids

During weightlessness and head-down body tilt, there is a redistribution of approximately 2 l of body fluids away from the dependent parts of the body and towards the head, neck, and thorax. This is caused by the decrease of the vein transmural pressure gradient as the value of $h\varrho G$ is now zero. For approximately 3 days the head and neck feel bloated, the neck veins are

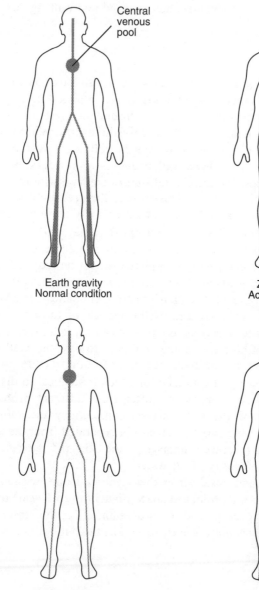

Central
venous
pool

Earth gravity
Normal condition

Zero gravity
Acute exposure

Zero gravity
Chronic exposure

Earth gravity
Upon return

Fig. 9.2. Diagram of the postulated mechanism of cardiovascular 'deconditioning' explained in the text. From Howard, P. (1982). In *Principles and Practice of Human Physiology* (ed. Edholm, O.G. and Weiner, J.S.). Academic Press, London.

engorged, and the legs become thinner (Fig. 9.2). During this period a diuresis takes place, initiated by increases in pressure in the volume receptors in the atria and great veins (Gauer–Henry reflex). A decrease in antidiuretic hormone and an increase in atrial natriuretic peptide secretion have been measured. This diuresis corrects the excess of fluid in the thoracic veins and so reduces the increased cardiac output and load on the heart due to excess venous return (Fig. 9.2). In water-immersion studies, these changes are enhanced, probably because water immersion compresses the interstitium.

Weightlessness causes the red and white blood cell counts to fall. Since cell breakdown does not change, this implies that production falls by more than the decrease in plasma volume that has just been described. Indeed, for an unknown reason bone marrow activity almost ceases, at least during the first days of weightlessness. The long-term effects of depressed immune responses in cosmonauts have still to be assessed.

9.3.3 The cardiovascular system

Initially, weightlessness causes an increase in cardiac output due to the lack of venous pooling. After correction of this (see above), cardiac output and heart rate fall. These changes are evidence of an adjustment of the cardio-vascular system to a zero-G environment. They are caused by a decreased sympathetic tone and increased parasympathetic tone and reflect the fact that the amount of work that must be performed by the heart has decreased. Some reports suggest that, with longer periods of weightlessness (over 50 days), a degree of ventricular atrophy occurs. This general 'decondition-ing' of the cardiovascular system under prolonged zero-G conditions can also be seen when the responses to circulatory 'stresses' are considered. Thus, the cardiovascular changes produced by exercise are more marked and, after experimentally decreasing venous return (for example, by inflat-ing cuffs around the thighs), the time that elapses before fainting occurs is decreased. The implications of these changes for cosmonauts returning to a gravitational field or bedridden patients starting to stand and walk again, will be considered later.

9.3.4 The central nervous system and muscles

A substantial proportion of cosmonauts experience giddiness, disorienta-tion, nausea, and even vomiting during the first few days in space. These symptoms are not observed during water immersion and bed-rest studies (thus showing the problems associated with extrapolation of data from indirect studies of weightlessness) and are attributed to an imbalance between different neural inputs to the brain. The input from the semi-circular canals (which reflects angular acceleration) is similar to that found on Earth, but inputs from skin, muscle and joint receptors (which signal the postural forces acting on the body), and the otolith receptors (which signal the orientation of the head in a gravitational field) change considerably. Similar problems can be produced on Earth by time spent on board ship (seasickness) and by prolonged rides at the fairground. Again abnormal vestibular inputs to the brain are implicated. Attempts to predict those cosmonauts in whom problems will be severe from experiments investigating vestibulo-ocular and optokinetic reflexes on Earth have so far been unsuccessful.

All objects, not just cosmonauts, are weightless in zero-G and yet their inertial properties are unchanged. For example, to hold a large hammer in a zero-G environment requires no effort, but to use it to strike an object requires the same force as on Earth. These 'abnormal' phenomena and the absence of a distinction between 'up' and 'down' require time for the necessary mental adjustment.

Movement is limited by lack of cabin space, which is sometimes a problem and there is far less need for tonic activity in 'antigravity' extensor muscles. As a result, muscular atrophy occurs as indicated by direct measures of strength and fatigue and by the increased excretion of urea in the urine.

Some studies have suggested that postural reflexes become exaggerated with continued weightlessness. The 'resetting' that this implies is similar to that described later (see Chapter 11) for the cardiovascular system in response to exercise.

9.3.5 The skeleton

All the changes in response to zero-G described so far reach equilibrium after a few weeks or months, when adjustment to weightlessness might be thought to be complete. However, demineralization of bones continues at an unchanged rate during 6 months of bed-rest or even during space flights of approximately 1 year (the longest time so far studied). This loss of bone material can be measured directly from densitometric studies of individual bones or indirectly from rates of urinary excretion of hydroxyproline and calcium. The bones most affected are those that normally bear the weight of the body. The rate of loss of minerals is approximately 0.5 per cent of the total per month: this implies a considerable danger of fractures on return to a normal, 1-G environment after approximately 2 years in space. The increased urinary calcium concentration might also increase the incidence of renal calculi, though this has not yet been found.

9.3.6 The return to Earth

We can conclude that, to a very considerable extent, we are able to adjust to a zero-G environment. The problem which remains is that of being able to withstand a gravitational field on return to Earth (or any other planet) or on standing up and beginning to walk again after being bedridden. The potential hazard from bone demineralization has been mentioned already, but other problems exist. On return to an upright posture, blood once again pools in the dependent parts of the body (Fig. 9.2). Bearing in mind that the blood volume is decreased by at least 10 per cent, that tissue tone might be reduced, and that a further 'resetting' of the vestibular reflexes is necessary (since fresh inputs from the otoliths and receptors involved in kinaesthesia are being sent to the central nervous system), the difficulties of standing upright become obvious. A decreased tolerance of the cardiovascular system to the stresses imposed by decreased venous return and exercise is observed immediately after the return to Earth.

In the days following their return, cosmonauts drink copiously, their kidneys conserve salt, and the number of circulating reticulocytes increases as the anaemia due to the previous low haemopoietic activity of the bone marrow is corrected. More slowly, cardiac muscle and skeletal muscle also recover. The rate of recovery has not been studied at all fully but it is essentially complete after 5 months and cosmonauts have undertaken subsequent flights without evidence of residual ill-effects from an earlier flight. The position is not as clear, however, with regard to the recalcification of bone. Recalcification is considerably slower than decalcification but there is no clear evidence that the osteoporosis is ever fully corrected. Moreover, the relative importance of bone formation and resorption, of calcitonin, vitamin D, and parathyroid hormone, and of changes to different types of bone, are all areas where adequate data have yet to be obtained.

9.3.7 Countermeasures

Much effort has gone into minimizing the unpleasant side-effects and the 'deconditioning' associated with prolonged weightlessness. Since nausea is most marked following head movement, some Russian cosmonauts have worn caps that restrict such movement. Methods aimed at opposing the process of 'deconditioning' have attempted to reproduce the normal orthostatic 'stresses' that occur when standing upright in a 1-G environment. The methods include a suction device applied around the legs and thighs that causes blood to be pooled in the legs and so decreases venous return, work schedules with a bicycle ergometer, springs, or isometric contractions, and the wearing of 'constant-load suits', which require the continuous expenditure of muscle effort. It must be realized that conventional training methods are often inadequate in a weightless environment where there is no weight to pull or push against. Exercise apparatus in weightless conditions, therefore, either requires the subject to be strapped into the device or has been designed so that one muscle group can pull against another.

Just before the cosmonauts return to Earth, extra measures are taken to prepare them for the increased G-forces associated with the deacceleration produced by re-entry into the Earth's atmosphere. For example, cosmonauts have worn 'antigravity suits' and have had their body fluid volume deliberately expanded by drinking saline.

Post-flight investigations indicate that these measures reduce the cardiovascular 'deconditioning' produced by space flight and decrease the problems after returning to Earth. However, the changes in erythropoiesis and vestibular function and the wasting of skeleton muscle, cardiac muscle, and bone wasting are by no means completely prevented. Furthermore, it is not known which type of countermeasure is best and to what degree and for how long it should be used. Anyway, increasing the duration and intensity of exercise becomes impracticable since it intrudes upon the cosmonauts' duties; the space available for exercise and the cosmonauts' motivation are also limiting factors. A basic problem is that, under terrestrial conditions, gravity exerts its effects continuously. To duplicate this in space would require the creation of an artificial gravity by imparting a spin (and, hence, centrifugal force) to the spacecraft. The size of centrifugal force needed to prevent 'deconditioning' is not known. Since the centrifugal force is proportional to the radius of rotation as well as angular velocity, if the force required to prevent 'deconditioning' is at all substantial, then the angular velocity of a small spacecraft (but not a large space station) might be unacceptably large to allow for navigation and routine manoeuvres. It is clear that much further work is needed to establish the most appropriate combination of countermeasures for cosmonauts whose stay in a zero-G environment is a prolonged one.

For bedridden patients such countermeasures are often inappropriate and so the process of deconditioning goes unchecked. It is necessary, therefore, for the patients to be strictly supervised and to undergo appropriate physiotherapy during their first days after getting up.

Further reading

Various authors (1984). *Science*, **225**, 205–34. (A series of papers reviewing Spacelab.)

Rambaut, P.C. and Goode, A.W. (1985). Skeletal changes during space flight. *Lancet*, **2**, 1050–2.

Various authors (1987). *Aviation, space and environmental medicine*, **58 Suppl.**, A1–A276. (Physiological adaptation of man in space.)

Various authors (1990). *Federation of American Societies of Experimental Biology (FASEB)*, **4**, 5–110. (Results from Cosmos biosatellites.)

10

Altered time

10.1 Basic concepts in chronobiology

We live in a rhythmic world. In most places on Earth there is an alternation between night and day. Because the Earth is tilted on its axis with respect to its plane of movement about the sun, the length of a day varies during the course of a year and gives rise to the seasons. Near the equator, such changes are modest; as one moves towards the poles, however, the changes become more marked. The seasons can be very different not only in the mean daily temperature but also in the distribution of light and darkness. In temperate latitudes, daylight can last as long as 16 h and as little as 8 h in the summer and winter respectively. Once the Arctic and Antarctic Circles have been reached, daylight can be non-existent during winter or continuous during summer.

In modern societies, we are not constrained by these forces. The invention of artificial lighting has allowed us, at least in theory, to choose our hours of sleep and leisure. In practice we are constrained by another set of time cues, those provided by our work and the society in which we live. Most of us live a life dominated by the '9-to-5' job and there are accepted regular times for shopping, eating, making less noise, etc. We have replaced the natural 24 h rhythms of our environment with artificial ones which synchronize us to a 24 h lifestyle in a way that is generally independent of the seasons.

10.1.1 Body time

Perhaps it is not surprising, therefore, that detailed measurements of physiological variables such as body temperature and heart rate show that these also have a daily rhythm related to our habits (Fig. 10.1). Most peak during the daytime and are at a minimum at night. Detailed examination of individuals over several days indicates that these rhythms are reliably present with a regular timing and period of exactly 24 h. This result could be construed as a reflection of our habits and environment, that is, a more light, noisy, and bustling environment when we are active in the daytime and a quieter and darker environment when we sleep at night.

10.1.2 Internal and external causes of body time

Two observations indicate that this is not fully correct. First, close examination of the temperature and blood pressure rhythms in Fig. 10.1 reveals falls in the evening before sleep and rises at the end of sleep before waking. That is, an anticipatory element seems to be present in the rhythms. Second, these rhythms do not disappear when a person maintains a constant routine for 24 h, that is, stays awake and sedentary and takes identical snacks regularly, in an environment in which noise, temperature, humidity, and lighting are kept constant (Fig. 10.2). This indicates that there must be an *internal* cause of the rhythm observed during this constant routine. In turn, this has given rise to the concept of an internal or body clock. Even so, our environment and habits do exert some effect. This is clearly shown by a comparison of the temperature rhythms observed during a constant routine and during the normal alternation between daytime activities and nocturnal sleep in a normal environment. These effects of normal habits are described as

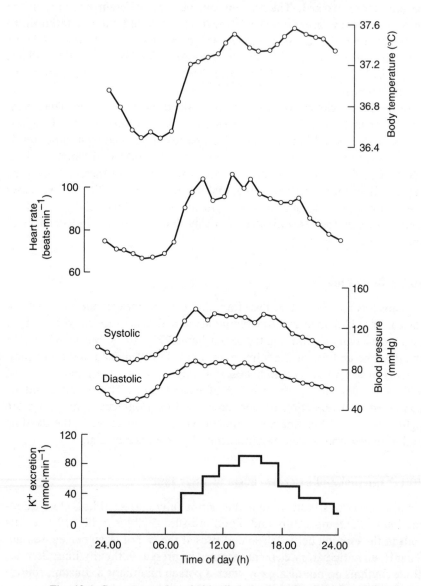

Fig. 10.1. Some examples of circadian rhythms from subjects who slept at night (0000–0800) and ate, drank, and were active during the day.

external, to distinguish them from those produced by the internal clock. Importantly, these two components, internal and external, are normally in phase, with the result that the changes mediated by the body clock are accentuated by those produced by our habits and environment.

10.1.3 Some properties of body time

To study body time in more detail, time cues from the outside environment must be removed. In this way, it is argued, any rhythmicity that remains must come from within the individual and so be a reflection of the internal clock. These are called free-running experiments. Early experiments required individuals to stay in underground caves; more recently, specially constructed isolation units have been used. What both types of experiment have shown is that rhythms do not die away or become erratic with time.

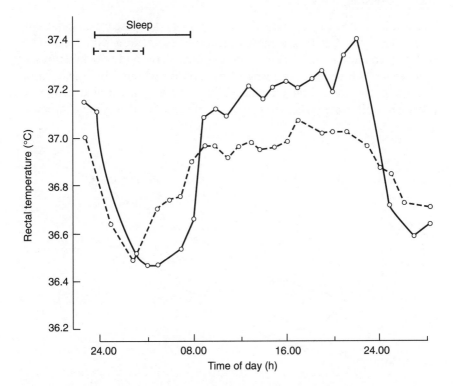

Fig. 10.2. Mean circadian changes in rectal temperature measured hourly in eight subjects living a normal nychthemeral existence (------) and in the same subjects during a constant routine in which they were woken at 0400 and spent the subsequent 24 h awake in a constant light and taking hourly small identical snacks (------). From Minors, D.S. and Waterhouse, J.M. (1981). *Circadian rhythms and the human.* John Wright, Bristol.

However, the free-running rhythm measured under these conditions does not have a cycle length of exactly 24 h but is slightly longer, approximately 25 h in humans (see Fig. 10.3). For this reason such a rhythm is called circadian (Latin: circa, about; diem, a day). The fact that the cycle length of the body clock differs from 24 h is very strong evidence for its origin being independent of the external environment.

Close inspection of Fig. 10.3 shows another result that is important. If the individual stayed awake longer than usual, as on day 6, for example, then sleep was *shorter* than usual as the waking time was not delayed by as great an amount. This suggests that the length of sleep is not determined by the amount of prior wakefulness but rather that waking tends to occur at a certain phase of the body clock—going to bed late means that this point is reached after a shorter amount of sleep.

10.1.4 Adjusting body time

The results of free-running experiments establish the presence of an internal clock. The fact that it is a poor timekeeper (compared with solar time) threatens to undermine its usefulness. In practice, the body clock is adjusted to an exact 24 h period (cycle length) by several rhythms from the environment and the individual's habits. These rhythms are called zeitgebers (German: Zeit, time; geber, to give). For many animals it is the alternation

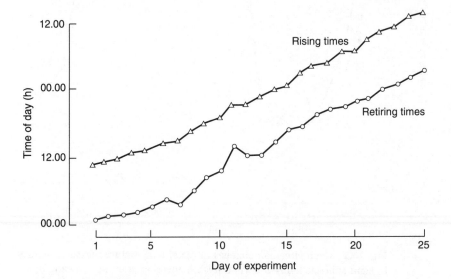

Fig. 10.3. Times of retiring and rising on successive occasions in an individual isolated from all knowledge of the passage of time, a free running experiment. From Waterhouse, J.M., Minors, D.S., and Waterhouse, M.E. (1990). *Your body clock*. Oxford University Press.

of light between day and night that acts as a zeitgeber. Indeed, our description of animals as 'nocturnal' or 'diurnal' acknowledges this. Other environmental influences, such as food availability and social cues, can also play a role, particularly in the interactions between parent and newborn offspring. In humans, natural lighting can adjust the body clock (as can artificial light of a sufficient intensity), but regular mealtimes, activity, and social influences are all effective to some degree. These 'alternative' zeitgebers are likely to be the dominant ones for many people who are rarely exposed to natural light, particularly during the winter or for the blind (see later). In practice, it is most useful to consider all potential time cues as providing a 'zeitgeber package' that continually adjusts the body clock; this will enable advice to be given (see later) to those who suffer problems because their lifestyle and body clock are not synchronized.

10.2 Some properties of the body clock

10.2.1 The site of the body clock

The site of the body clock has been the subject of much research, necessarily conducted upon animals. There is now a very large amount of data which points to the hypothalamic paired suprachiasmatic nuclei (SCN) as being a crucial part of the internal timing system. The main lines of evidence are the following.

1. The SCN show a circadian rhythm of uptake of the non-metabolized glucose analogue, 2-deoxy-D-glucose.

2. The rate of firing of neurones in the SCN continues to show a circadian rhythm when the SCN have been separated from the rest of the CNS by surgery (Fig. 10.4). This indicates that a neural input to the SCN is not necessary for them to be rhythmic (see point 1 above).

3. Slices of SCN incubated *in vitro* show circadian rhythms of neuronal firing frequency and release of neurotransmitter. This result removes the possibility that humoral factors accounted for the rhythm in point 2 above.

4. Removal of the SCN generally leads to a loss of circadian rhythmic activity or drinking in the animal. This rhythmicity can be recovered if cells from the hypothalamus containing the germinal areas for the SCN are transplanted back into the animal from a fetus. Moreover, if material from a fetus with a mutant clock period is used (that is, an animal that, when adult, will show a rhythm that is abnormally rapid or slow) then the rhythm that develops in the host shows the mutant period. This last point indicates that the clock itself, a structure able to generate a *particular periodicity*—rather

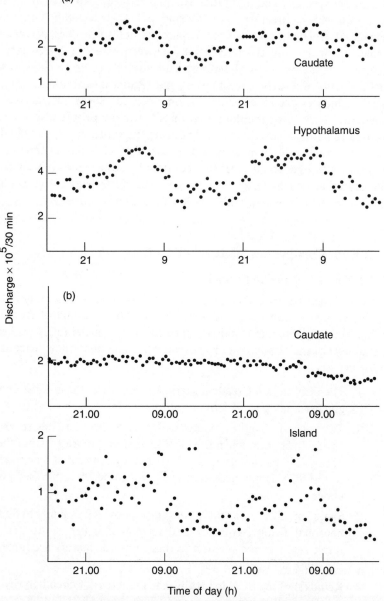

Fig. 10.4. Circadian rhythm of neuronal activity before and after isolation of the hypothalamus. In an intact rat (a), multiple unit activity has a circadian rhythm both in hypothalamic and caudate regions. After the hypothalamus was isolated by knife cuts (b), recordings from within the hypothalamic island indicated persisting rhythmicity, while no rhythmicity was evident outside the island, thus suggesting the presence of a hypothalamic circadian pacemaker. From Inouye, S. and Kawamura, H. (1979). *Proc. Nat. Acad. Sci. USA*, **76**, 5961.

than some structure able to produce a generalized rhythmicity—has been transplanted.

10.2.2 The pineal gland—part of the body clock?

There is also evidence that the pineal gland, a structure in the roof of the midbrain that secretes the indoleamine, melatonin, plays some part in generating and controlling body time. In birds and other animals which show seasonal rhythms (migration or breeding, for example), the pineal gland is an important link between changes in the external environment and the many biochemical and physiological changes they evoke. In humans, such seasonal changes appear to be unimportant, but this additional link between rhythmicity in the environment and the body might remain and add to the accuracy of phase control of the body clock. Receptors for melatonin are present in the SCN and this would support the view that some functional connection exists. This evidence, and that summarized in the next section, leads to the current view that the SCN and pineal gland interact to form the body clock.

10.2.3 How zeitgebers work

The means by which zeitgebers act also point to the SCN and pineal having complementary roles. An anatomical link between the retina and the SCN, the retinohypothalamic tract, has been found. This carries information about mean light intensity to the SCN. Other work has shown that a pulse of bright light given to hamsters kept in constant dark can adjust the body clock, the amount and direction of adjustment depending upon the time when the bright light is given.

A similar response has also been observed recently in humans. Bright light at the end of the night, just after the minimum rectal temperature has been reached, tends to advance the body clock. Bright light at the beginning of the night and just before the temperature minimum is reached tends to delay it. In the middle of the day bright light has no effect. Melatonin is normally secreted in the late evening and at night and is suppressed by bright light. Ingestion of this hormone also appears to produce shifts of the body clock; evening doses advance it and morning ones delay it. In other words, melatonin secretion has the opposite effect to bright light. In practice, therefore, bright light in the morning advances the body clock not only via the retinohypothalamic tract but also because it suppresses melatonin secretion. Similarly, bright light in the evening delays the body clock by both mechanisms. As a result the circadian body clock can be adjusted to an exact 24 h period; in the morning any delay of the clock will result in the zeitgebers inducing advances and in the evening, light will delay it.

The means by which social and physical activities and mealtimes might act as zeitgebers is less well known. Even so, this lack of information about detailed mechanisms need not negate their value as potential zeitgebers.

10.3 The significance of circadian rhythms

10.3.1 The usefulness of circadian rhythms

What use is served by circadian rhythms? Briefly, they enable regular environmental changes to be predicted. They are, therefore fundamentally different from homeostatic mechanisms that respond *after* the event to changes produced in the body by the environment. Thus, plasma adrenalin concentration and body temperature both rise before waking, preparing us for the rigours of a new day and these variables fall in the evening, preparing us for relaxation and sleep. Such changes, produced by the body clock, are independent of the external environment. It appears that the output from the body clock can change the sensitivity and threshold of various elements in a feedback loop. For example, sweating and cutaneous vasodilatation are initiated at lower temperatures during the night than the day. As a result, the set-point of the thermoregulatory system shows circadian variation, with body temperature being *controlled* at a higher value during the daytime than the night.

Homeostatic control loops also receive advance warning of impending changes before the variable they control actually deviates from its set-point. This warning input is provided by 'disturbance detectors' which are 'outside' the feedback loop (unlike the misalignment detectors which are part of the loop itself). An example would be presence of cutaneous thermo-receptors which initiate shivering when a person enters a cold environment before any change occurs in deep body temperature.

Clearly this combination of feedback loops, disturbance detectors, and the body clock enables a person to respond to changes in the environment as well as to act independently of them. The body as a whole responds because the major rhythmic outputs of the body clock, those of body temperature, plasma adrenalin, and other hormones, exert their effects very widely. We are rhythmic creatures who live in a rhythmic world.

10.3.2 Problems associated with circadian rhythms

10.3.2.1 *Jet lag and time-zone transitions*

Another important property of the circadian system is its stability, that is, its resistance to rapid change. The advantage of this is that a daytime nap or a nightime snack does not cause the body clock to shift. Whilst the evolutionary advantage of this is clear, it causes difficulties for those who fly long distances across several time zones and for those who are required to work at night.

For several days after flying across several time zones, people feel tired during part of the day and yet cannot achieve a full night's sleep. They feel irritable, lose their appetite, have irregular bowel movements, and lose their powers of concentration. In brief, they feel 'below par' and are suffering from 'jet lag'. The severity of the symptoms is proportional to the number of time zones crossed and is generally worse and lasts longer after a flight to the east compared with one to the west.

The symptoms arise because, for some days after the flight, the body clock remains adjusted to the time zone the traveller has just left. Objective measurements of mental performance, cortisol secretion, and deep body temperature (Fig. 10.5), for example, confirm this delay in adjustment. As a result, there is a mismatching between the internal and external components of the rhythms. In accord with this explanation is the observation that north–south flights produce the same amounts of stress and fatigue as do transmeridian ones, but they do not produce jet lag.

Resetting the body clock takes place over the subsequent days due to the action of the new local zeitgebers. It should be remembered that the clock's natural period is approximately 25 h. Therefore, adjustment to eastward flights is more difficult than to westward flights (and, hence, jet lag is worse) because the body clock must be advanced rather than delayed. For the same reason, flights which cross 12 time zones are generally associated with delays, not advances, of the body clock.

Jet lag can be mitigated either by combating the symptoms directly or by promoting adjustment of the body clock. Sleep difficulties can be alleviated by the use of a hypnotic such as a short-acting benzodiazepine. Several ways of promoting adjustment of the body clock have been suggested, generally involving one or more of the zeitgebers that are believed normally to be important. Such an approach might entail a full and regular adjustment of lifestyle (for example, mealtimes) in the new time zone and, in particular, exposure at the appropriate time to natural light. Bearing in mind that bright light immediately after the temperature minimum tends to advance the clock and before it tends to delay the clock, a protocol for the appropriate times both to seek and to avoid bright light can be devised (see Table 10.1). Thus, in the days immediately after a flight to the east across eight time zones (for example, from the UK to Japan), exposure to bright light is recommended between 1300 and 1900 local time (0500 and 1100 by unadjusted body time) and should be avoided between 0500 and 1100 local time (2100 and 0300 body time) since this would tend to *delay* the body clock.

It is known that melatonin capsules taken in the afternoon or evening (local time) reduce the fatigue associated with jet lag. It is likely that this effect is achieved through an adjustment of the body clock. The possible interaction between the pineal gland and the SCN via light has also been described already.

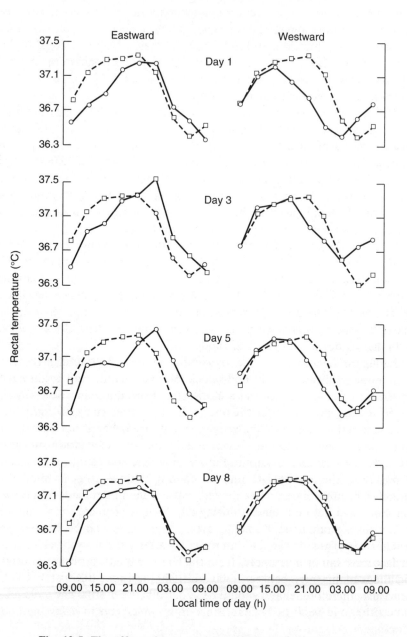

Fig. 10.5. The effect of transmeridian flight through six time zones in an eastward or westward direction upon the rhythm of rectal temperature. Pre-flight data (□----□), represented for clarity on each post-flight day. Post-flight data (○——○). Data represent the means from eight subjects. From Klein, K.E., Wegmann, H-M., and Hunt, B.I. (1972). *Aerospace Med.*, **43**, 119.

Table 10.1. Appropriate times to seek and avoid bright light. From Waterhouse, J.M., Minors, D.S. and Waterhouse, M.E.(1990) *Your body clock*. Oxford University Press, Oxford.

	Bad local times for exposure to natural light	Good local times for exposure to natural light
Time zones to the west		
4 h	0100–0700*	1700–2300†
8 h	2100–0300*	1300–1900†
12 h	1700–2300*	0900–1500†
Time zones to the east		
4 h	0100–0700†	0900–1500*
8 h	0500–1100†	1300–1900*
12 h	Treat this as 12 hours to the west	

* This will tend to advance the body clock.
† This will tend to delay the body clock.

10.3.2.2 Shift work

Working at night, when we are at the trough of our circadian rhythms of body temperature, alertness, and mental and physical performance, and sleeping during the daytime, when body temperature, urine production, and plasma adrenalin are all high, are other circumstances in which the body clock is something of a disadvantage. Some of the problems of shift work are similar to those after time-zone transitions. For example, the work pattern, whether rotating shifts or permanent night shifts, is continually changing between 'abnormal' work times and normal work times or rest days. As a result, the shift worker is in a similar position to a traveller forever jet-setting around the globe. However, there are important differences. First, night work might occupy many years of a person's working life. Second, it will be associated with poorer mental and physical performance in circumstances where public safety is at stake (air traffic controllers and nuclear power station workers are obvious examples). Finally and perhaps most importantly, there is a clash between the shift worker's habits and those of his/her spouse, family and close friends. It is perhaps not surprising, therefore, that some find the demands and problems too great and choose to leave night work. More worryingly, the incidences of gastro-intestinal ulcers, chronic fatigue, and cardiovascular disorders are all raised in comparison with a matched sample of people working only during the daytime. The exact role played by the circadian timing system in causing these problems is not certain though difficulties with daytime sleep and fatigue and poorer performance during the work period, are obvious results. Proposed solutions, based upon strengthening zeitgebers, are often unacceptable. For example, the advice to adjust one's habits as fully as possible to a night-work/day-sleep schedule is socially unacceptable to the majority of those with families. The body clock and night work are uneasy bedfellows and those involved and society at large, have to pay a social and medical cost.

10.3.3 Circadian rhythms in clinical practice

10.3.3.1 *Abnormal body clocks*

The above problems arise because we impose upon ourselves an unnatural lifestyle. However, problems can also arise due to a malfunction of the body clock. Cases in which the circadian rhythms are apparently not adjusted to the 24 h day have been reported (Fig. 10.6). This causes obvious difficulties with sleeping at night and feeling alert during the day and is associated with mild depression. Such a disorder is not uncommon in blind people, in whom there is obviously an inability to respond to light as a zeitgeber, but it has been reported in sighted individuals also, particularly if they ignore conventional zeitgebers. Less extreme and therefore more common, are cases in which adjustment of the body clock to the solar day exists, but is poor. This abnormality manifests itself as temporary bouts of insomnia or fatigue. These might reflect a poorly adjusted body clock, but a rather erratic lifestyle with respect to mealtimes and hours of sleep and activity is often the cause, rather than the result, of an inaccurate body clock. A further type of abnormality is termed Delayed Sleep Phase Syndrome. As its name suggests, the sufferer can sleep regularly, but only at times that are much later than normal (about 0400–1200). In practice this becomes incompatible with a conventional occupation and chronic sleep loss results also.

All these abnormalities result from some inadequacy in the processes by which zeitgebers entrain the body clock; the error might be in the zeitgebers (or lack of them) themselves or in the clock. In all cases, some alleviation of the problem is produced by strengthening zeitgebers; regular times of sleep, meals, and bouts of exercise have all had some success. Interestingly, the ingestion of melatonin capsules each evening has also been shown to be useful. It is not yet clear if this is due to the action of this hormone upon the SCN.

All rhythms, including those of the sleep/wake cycle, hormones, and body temperature are affected equally in these disorders. By contrast, there is an uncommon form of endogenous depression in which the circadian rhythms appear to be dissociated from one another. That is, even though the times of sleep are not particularly abnormal, other rhythms, such as body temperature and plasma melatonin and cortisol, are phased abnormally early or late or erratically. This disorder is much more common in wintertime (and is therefore called Seasonal Affective Disorder) and in-

Time of day (h)

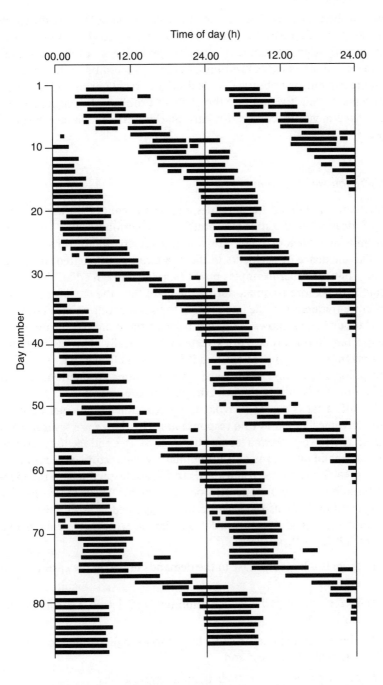

Fig. 10.6. An example of a sighted individual in which sleep times (shown as the bars) are not adjusted to the 24 h day. From Kokkoris, C.P., Weitzman, E.D., Pollock, G.P., Spielman, A.J., Czeisler, C.A., and Bradlow, H. (1978). *Sleep*, **1**, 177.

creases in incidence and the nearer one lives to the poles. Treatment with bright artificial light is often successful. It is claimed that the bright light works by adjusting the timing of rhythms (so acting as a zeitgeber) and for this reason it is given in the morning or evening according to the direction in which the rhythms are observed to be displaced from normal. However, this claim remains tentative because the difficult problem of devising a suitable control treatment, to correct for any placebo effect, has not been fully solved.

10.3.3.2 *Non-elective events*

Accidents in the home, the time of spontaneous childbirth, and the incidence of deaths from asthmatic attacks and cardiovascular emergencies (ischaemia and haemorrhage) are not distributed evenly throughout the 24 h. The incidence of accidents in the home can be attributed to our daily routines, but the other examples might be related to circadian rhythmicity.

Childbirth is more frequent during the night than the day because labour starts more frequently in the late evening than at any other time. The time at which labour begins shows a rhythm because the maternal hormones that are important in this process are secreted rhythmically. The fetus too might be important in initiating labour and it is well established that several daily rhythms, including those of movement and hormone production, are manifested by the fetus during the last trimester of pregnancy.

Asthmatic attacks can be provoked by environmental allergens but there is also a greater likelihood of a response at night. There are several reasons for this: the lowest plasma concentrations of the endogenous bronchodilator adrenalin and of the anti-inflammatory agent cortisol occur at night and the greatest tendency of mast cells to release histamine and the highest vagal bronchoconstrictor tone also occur at night. These mechanisms are present in all individuals but seem to be exaggerated in asthmatics.

An increased incidence of cardiovascular emergencies occurs between 0600 and 1200. At these times:

(1) there is a large increase in the demands made on the cardiovascular system;

(2) increased sympathetic activation tends to decrease coronary blood flow;

(3) blood pressure rises from its lowest to its highest value so producing mechanical stresses; and

(4) blood platelets show their highest aggregability.

Though correlation is not proof of causality, it is widely suggested that this combination of factors will tend to increase the likelihood of haemorrhage, ischaemia, and related disorders.

10.3.3.3 *Clinical diagnosis*

As an aid to diagnosis, clinicians often wish to assess if some variable is increased or decreased in comparison with normal values. A knowledge of circadian rhythmicity can be important, since it enables a time to be chosen when an abnormality would be most clearly manifest. Consider the following examples (where the comments in brackets indicate the timing of the rhythm in health).

1. Growth hormone deficit is assessed during the first part of sleep (growth hormone normally peaks early in sleep, Fig. 10.7).
2. Cushing's syndrome is diagnosed in the evening (minimum cortisol secretion is just before sleep, Fig. 10.7).
3. Rheumatoid arthritis is worst in the morning (the anti-inflammatory action of cortisol in the joints is lowest in the morning and so stiffness, pain, and swelling are most marked then).
4. Fetal inactivity, indicative of distress, is best assessed in the evening (fetal movement is normally greater in the evening).
5. Decreased peak expiratory flow as an indicator of asthma is most clearly assessed early morning or late evening (for reasons considered above).

10.3.3.4 *Treatment*

The timing of treatment might also be important in some cases. As examples consider the following: for asthmatics, an inhaler containing a β-agonist should be readily available during the night and, if anti-inflammatory drugs are being used, the overnight plasma concentration should be maintained; for those suffering from rheumatoid arthritis, early morning also is again the time when sufficient anti-inflammatory activity should be present in the joints; for those with hypertension, the marked rise in blood pressure around the hours of waking should be minimized by ensuring adequate amounts of the antihypertensive drug in the plasma at this time.

A rather different example is provided by heparin, an anticoagulant that is often infused for extended periods to reduce the chance of thrombosis. Conventionally, a continuous infusion at a constant rate is given so that plasma concentrations are constant throughout the 24 h. This might not be the ideal arrangement because, as already mentioned, the tendency for platelet aggregation is highest immediately after waking and decreases throughout the daytime. Thus, a constant plasma concentration of heparin which is inadequate to reduce sufficiently the risk of blood clotting in

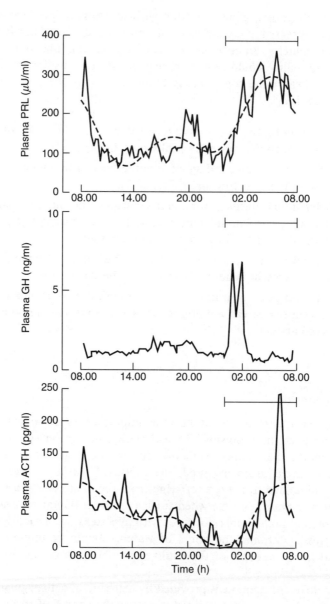

Fig. 10.7. Profiles (24 h) of plasma prolactin (PRL), growth hormone (GH), and corticotropin (ACTH) obtained simultaneously in a single subject. The sampling interval is 15 min. For PRL and ACTH, a best-fit curve quantifying the circadian waveshape is shown in dashed line. The black bars represent the sleep period. From Van Cauter, E. (1989). In Arendt, J., Minors, D.S. and Waterhouse, J.M. (ed.). *Biological rhythms in clinical practice.* Butterworth, Guildford.

the early morning has too great a chance of causing haemorrhage in the evening.

As a final example, consider hormone replacement therapy, treatment of delayed puberty, or injection of growth hormone due to inadequate secretion by the pituitary gland. Continuous infusions are rather ineffective because the target tissue becomes refractory to the secretagogue. Multiple-dose infusions are more effective, most of the dose being given at a time when the peak concentration of the hormone occurs normally (early morning for cortisol, night for growth hormone and gonadotrophins, see Fig. 10.7).

10.3.3.5 *Chronopharmacology*

The effectiveness of a given dose of drug can also vary with the time it is given. This phenomenon of chronotherapeutics has two components: chronopharmacokinetics and chronesthesy. Pharmacokinetics refers to the uptake, distribution, metabolism, and elimination of a drug. Many drugs are taken up from the gut and metabolized more quickly in the morning than in the evening. As a result, the profile of the plasma concentration rises and falls more quickly after morning administration. This has important consequences if it is necessary to maintain plasma concentrations of the drug within prescribed limits. Several factors contribute to this phenomenon, amongst which are gut blood flow and food content, the detoxifying activity of hepatic enzymes, and renal clearance.

Even if the plasma concentration of a drug is kept constant by intravenous infusion, the effect of the drug might vary with time, the phenomenon of chronesthesy. Although the reason is not well established, there is evidence that receptor number and affinity can show circadian rhythmicity. Whatever the reason, it is clear that conventional advice for taking drugs—'three times a day with meals', 'on rising and retiring'—might not be the most satisfactory.

Finally, let us consider the toxic side-effects produced by a drug. Normally these are not dose-limiting factors since the toxic dose is far greater than the therapeutic dose. With chronic drug administration and cancer chemotherapy, however, toxicity might become a major consideration. Cisplatin is an antimetabolite that is used in cancer chemotherapy whose side-effects include renal and bone marrow damage. Renal damage is lessened if the urine flow is high (because the concentration of the drug in the tubule is lessened). It is known that the renal responses to water- and saline-loading show a circadian rhythm, with peak diuresis and natriuresis occurring in the late afternoon rather than the early morning. Accordingly, cisplatin is less toxic when given at 1800 than at 0600 and so the treatment is more likely to be completed and to have a successful outcome.

Further reading

Arendt, J., Minors, D.S., and Waterhouse, J.M. (ed.) (1989). *Biological rhythms and clinical practice*. Butterworths, Guildford, UK.

Minors, D.S. and Waterhouse, J.M. (1981). *Circadian rhythms and the human*. John Wright, Bristol, UK.

Waterhouse, J.M., Minors, D.S., and Waterhouse, M.E. (1990). *Your body clock*. Oxford University Press.

11

Exercise

11.1 Introduction

11.1.1 Exercise

Exercise is a part of everyday life and needs the same kind (if not the same scale) of physiological adjustments as running a marathon. Formal exercise on a squash court, a running track, or a laboratory treadmill is just an extension of normal activity. To the physiologist, it is a natural way of applying stress to the body's homeostatic mechanisms. Although something can be learned about such mechanisms by observing them in a state of equilibrium, far more can be learned by deliberately disturbing that state and watching them readjust to a new equilibrium.

Nobody has an infinite capacity for exercise. What sets the limit? This is not normally an easy question to answer, since the physiological processes that co-operate to supply energy are well matched. However, in a patient with a cardiorespiratory disorder (who may show little distress at rest), even trivial exercise may expose a weak link quite dramatically. Thus, exercise can be useful clinically, in arriving at a diagnosis and in assessing both severity of disability and subsequent rehabilitation.

In this chapter, given values generally apply to young adults who are healthy, but not highly athletic and probably male. The main quantitative differences in females appear to follow from, on average, a smaller total muscle mass and a lower haemoglobin concentration in blood.

11.1.2 Types of exercise

It is useful to classify exercise in terms of the physiological adjustments it requires. For example, static ('isometric') exercise such as weightlifting is quite different from dynamic exercise such as rowing. Though similar muscle groups may be active in both, the patterns of contraction, of energy consumption, and of blood flow, are not the same.

Prolonged static exertion is uncommon (unless maintenance of posture is included), but both short spurts and sustained flows of energy are used in most forms of physical activity. The former are supplied largely from reserves within the muscles and generated by anaerobic processes (that is, ones which do not rely upon availability of oxygen). Since the time span is brief, there is little scope for cardiorespiratory adjustments during the exercise itself, though there may be anticipatory changes and there will be retrospective changes. On the other hand, a sustained flow of energy can be generated only by aerobic processes, which rely upon imported oxygen (and, eventually, oxidizable substrates). The rate at which oxygen can be supplied depends upon successful cardiorespiratory adaptation to the increased demand and may limit the rate at which energy can be generated. Broadly speaking, anaerobic sources can supply a limited quantity of energy at an unlimited rate, whereas aerobic sources can supply an unlimited quantity at a limited rate. Ultimately, energy drawn from anaerobic reserves must be replenished from aerobic sources.

The two forms of exercise and of energy supply are not mutually exclusive. Most everyday or athletic activities incorporate some features of both static and dynamic exercise and use different blends of aerobic and anaerobic energy at different stages of the activity. This is discussed in more detail in later sections (see pp. 246 and 255). First, we shall deal with dynamic 'steady-state' exercise, that is, where exercise continues at a steady pace within the capacity to generate energy aerobically and an equilibrium is reached between consumption of oxygen in the muscles and uptake of oxygen at the lungs.

11.2 Sources of energy

11.2.1. Adenosine triphosphate (ATP) and its regeneration

When cross-bridges are formed between actin and myosin in the course of muscular contraction, the high-energy compound ATP is hydrolysed to adenosine diphosphate (ADP) and inorganic phosphate (Pi). Under aerobic conditions, ATP can be resynthesized from ADP and Pi by oxidative phosphorylation. Alternatively, ADP can be rephosphorylated to ATP by transfer of a phosphate group from other high-energy compounds such as creatine phosphate or by substrate-level phosphorylation during glycolysis. Transfer from creatine phosphate is just an 'internal loan' and there is no net gain of high-energy compounds; its role is discussed later under anaerobic energy sources (p. 247). Substrate-level phosphorylation does result in a net gain and since it does not rely directly upon the presence of oxygen, can also take place anaerobically.

11.2.2 Pathways of energy production

The pathways involved in ATP synthesis are summarized in Fig. 11.1. Both carbohydrate and fat are used as substrates for energy production in skeletal and cardiac muscle. The relative amounts used vary with availability of the substrates, type of muscle, muscular activity, and supply of oxygen. In resting muscle and in muscles which are active over long periods (such as 'red' skeletal and cardiac muscle), fat is the major substrate under aerobic conditions.

Under aerobic conditions, the overall yield is 16 ATP molecules per 2-carbon unit of a fatty acid and 38 ATP per molecule of glucose or 39 ATP per molecule of glucose-6-phosphate derived from glycogen.

Under anaerobic conditions, glycolysis halts at pyruvate. However, the accumulating pyruvate can be reduced to lactate (much of which enters the blood) thereby oxidizing $NADH.H^+$ to NAD^+. Though no ATP results from this reaction, it does permit glycolysis to continue, yielding a net three ATP per molecule of glucose-6-phosphate. The usefulness of this grossly uneconomic reaction is discussed later under anaerobic energy sources (see p. 246). Fat, on the other hand, cannot be used as a substrate under anaerobic conditions.

11.2.3 Control of energy production

Physiologically, supplies of oxygen and substrates are the principal limitations upon aerobic production of ATP. Biochemically, the rate of oxidative phosphorylation is determined by the supply of ADP and Pi, which in turn reflects the rate at which ATP is used. The only limitation is the mitochondrial capacity for oxidative phosphorylation. This capacity is greatest in cardiac muscle and least in 'white' skeletal muscles which, typically, are active in short bursts and maximal efforts. The latter have a higher glycogenolytic capacity.

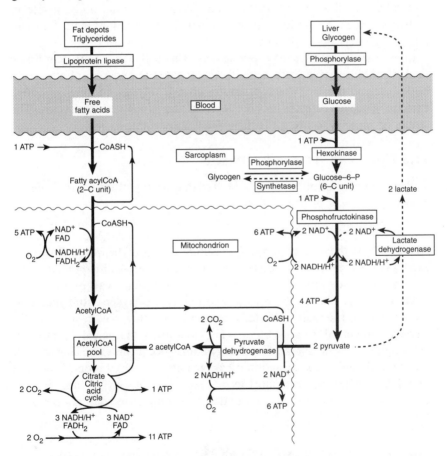

Fig. 11.1. Pathways of energy production in muscle. Only the principal regulatory (rate-limiting) enzymes are included. Alternative pathways are shown in broken lines.

In general, the extent to which a muscle uses fat parallels its capacity for oxidative phosphorylation and, hence, its mitochondrial density. Energy production from carbohydrate can be regarded as an 'optional extra', used to supplement the supply from fat as required. Its advantages are that the large intramuscular stores of glycogen can be used as a substrate at short notice and that a limited amount of energy can be supplied anaerobically. Its disadvantages are that it uses a scarce resource and that anaerobic glycolysis is wasteful of energy, even when lactate is recycled.

The principal internal controls act through product inhibition of key enzymes. For example, phosphofructokinase is inhibited by citrate and pyruvate dehydrogenase by acetyl coenzyme A; both are inhibited by ATP. Thus, when oxidation of fat is already generating sufficient acetyl CoA and ATP, glycolysis is suppressed. Phosphorylase is inhibited by glucose-6-phosphate and by ATP, so that glycogenolysis is suppressed when glucose and ATP supplies are adequate. Under anaerobic conditions, a rise in hydrogen ion concentration (resulting from accumulation of lactate) has an inhibitory effect upon glycolysis.

In exercise, adrenalin may be released. This activates lipoprotein lipase (which mobilizes free fatty acids from fat depots) and phosphorylase in both liver and muscle (which promotes glycogenolysis). In long-continued exercise, glycogen reserves become depleted and hypoglycaemia occurs. The ability of muscles to use fat is then vitally important.

11.3 Uptake of oxygen by muscle

The oxygen consumption of muscle, like that of any other tissue, is determined by the Fick principle, that is,

$$\dot{V}O_2 = \dot{Q} \times \Delta avO_2$$

where $\dot{V}O_2$ is the rate of oxygen consumption, $\dot{Q}$ is the blood flow, and ΔavO_2 is the arteriovenous difference of O_2 content. An increase in blood flow alone is an uneconomic and largely ineffective way of increasing oxygen supply. Unless the muscle extracts more oxygen from incoming arterial blood, the main result of a greater blood flow will be a rise in the oxygen content of venous blood. The solution is a typical example of autoregulation: the metabolic changes that occur in exercising muscle induce both increased extraction of oxygen and increased blood flow. The principles governing this short-term regulation of oxygen delivery are essentially the same as those that underlie the long-term adaptation seen at high altitude (see Chapter 7).

11.3.1 Extraction of oxygen from blood

Transfer of oxygen from blood in muscle capillaries to mitochondria within muscle cells occurs by diffusion. The factors which affect the rate of diffusion of a gas between blood and tissue cells (or in the lungs, between air and blood) are summarized by Fick's law of diffusion (not to be confused with Fick's principle, above).

Rate of diffusion =
(solubility/molecular weight) $\times$ (area/distance) $\times$ $(P_1 - P_2)$

where solubility and molecular weight are characteristics of the gas, area (available for diffusion) and distance (over which diffusion must occur) are characteristics of the vascular structure of the tissue, P_1 is the partial pressure of gas at the source (the capillary blood), and P_2 is the partial pressure of gas at the destination (the mitochondria).

The steeper the gradient of partial pressure of oxygen from blood to tissue, the faster the diffusion. The main variables affecting this gradient are the partial pressure of oxygen (PO_2) in capillary blood, the PO_2 in the mitochondria, and the distance oxygen must diffuse. The PO_2 in the capillary blood is initially that of arterial blood, but falls towards that in venous blood as the blood passes along the capillary. At rest the PO_2 in mitochondria is close to that in the venous blood from the muscle, that is, 20–30 mmHg (3–4 kPa). However, during exercise it may fall to 1 mmHg (0.15 kPa) before mitochondrial activity is impaired. This in itself makes the gradient of PO_2 steeper and speeds diffusion of oxygen from blood, that is, the demand accelerates the supply. The presence of myoglobin, in greater concentration in 'red' muscles, also assists diffusion within muscle.

Haemoglobin in venous blood from resting muscle is 40–60 per cent saturated with oxygen but in maximal exercise saturation falls to 15 per cent or less. This greater desaturation reflects a lower venous PO_2 of approximately 15 mmHg (2 kPa) and also a displacement of the oxyhaemoglobin dissociation curve to the right by products of metabolism such as CO_2, H^+, and heat. In femoral venous blood of a trained subject, P_{50} at rest was 26 mmHg (3.5 kPa) but rose to 39 mmHg (5.2 kPa) during maximal leg exercise. PO_2 fell to 10 mmHg (1.3 kPa) and saturation to 5 per cent. Thus, in maximal exercise, ΔavO_2 can be twice that at rest.

It follows that, during maximal exercise, oxygen is diffusing from blood to muscle at least twice as fast as at rest, despite a lower capillary PO_2. In part, this results from the fall in PO_2 of the tissues (above), but the third component of the diffusion gradient (the distance) also changes; so does the area of capillary wall. These (the distance and area) depend on the distribution of blood flow in the capillary network.

11.3.2 Blood flow in muscle

In resting muscle, tonic sympathetic nervous activity constricts arterioles and reduces blood flow to 20–30 ml/min/kg. The distribution of this flow within the microcirculation is controlled by the opening and closing of precapillary sphincters in response to local metabolism. At rest the majority of sphincters are closed and most of the flow is confined to main or 'thorough-fare' channels, so that effective capillary density is probably approximately 100 mm^{-2}.

In working muscles, PO_2 falls, whereas the partial pressure of carbon dioxide (PCO_2), temperature, osmotic activity, and the concentrations of H$^+$, K$^+$, and ADP in interstitial fluid all rise. These local factors relax pre-capillary sphincters and override the centrally controlled vasoconstriction of the arterioles. Some selective sympathetic vasodilatation may also occur. As a result of the reduced resistance, total blood flow rises towards a maximum of approximately 500 ml/min/kg. Relaxation of the sphincters and the rise of perfusion pressure open dormant capillaries: estimates of capillary density in human quadriceps femoris during maximal exercise are in the range 300–700 mm^{-2}. The greater total flow is therefore spread more evenly across a larger number of capillaries. Since the flow has increased 20-fold and the number of patent capillaries approximately five-fold, the flow rate through individual capillaries must be more rapid than at rest. On the other hand, the distance the oxygen must diffuse is now shorter and the area of the capillary walls has increased; diffusion is more rapid and the blood is efficiently desaturated before it leaves the capillary. Overall, then, total oxygen uptake by muscle has increased 40-fold. There are also changes in fluid balance across the capillary wall (see p. 254).

Local metabolic events in exercising muscle enhance blood flow, but the mechanical events tend to impede it. During a vigorous contraction, intra-muscular pressure can rise far above systolic arterial pressure and flow ceases. This is a major problem in static exercise (see p. 246), but in rhyth-mic dynamic exercise, the subsequent relaxation of the muscle allows blood flow to resume. Thus, flow occurs in spurts between contractions.

11.3.3 Implications for peripheral circulation

Skeletal muscle constitutes 40–45 per cent of lean body mass. At rest, it receives less than 20 per cent of the cardiac output but, if maximally active, it would require 300–400 per cent. Clearly, if no compensatory action were taken to meet the increased demand for blood flow, arterial blood pressure would fall. In practice, an initial fall of blood pressure does not occur because anticipatory mechanisms forestall it (see p. 248). For the present, we will ignore these and suppose that a fall has occurred and that corrections have been initiated through the baroreceptor reflex pathway.

An obvious response is an increase in cardiac output to match the in-creased demand. However, this cannot be achieved instantaneously because it requires an increased venous return (see p. 239). More immediately useful is a generalized vasoconstriction resulting from increased sympathetic activity. Some tissues are spared, namely the high-priority circulations of brain and heart which are permanently protected against outside interference and the working muscles where local metabolic factors predominate. Other tissues have no such protection: the principal victims are the splanchnic (gut and liver) and renal circulations (where blood flow in maximal exercise can be as low as 30 per cent of normal), the skin, and non-working muscles. The net result is that up to half of the resting cardiac output can be diverted away from these tissues towards the working muscles: this is equivalent to a three-fold increase in total muscle blood flow. This may seem a small gain, which could not be maintained without damage to the vasoconstricted organs. Even so, it is useful in bridging the gap before cardiac output rises and in ensuring that none of the increase in cardiac output, when it does occur, is wasted upon these (temporarily) irrelevant organs. Blood flow to skin may later rise again if body temperature increases (see p. 254).

11.4 Cardiac output

The heart meets the demands of the tissues for blood flow; it does not impose flow upon them. This service is provided by adjusting cardiac output to maintain a sufficient perfusion pressure irrespective of the total peripheral resistance. A small or temporary increase in demand by one tissue may be compensated for by constriction elsewhere, so that the total resistance is unaltered. A large, continued increase in demand necessitates an increase in cardiac output. However, the heart cannot sustain a greater output until it receives a greater input. A rise in heart rate, alone, may increase left heart output for a few beats by drawing upon blood in the pulmonary veins, but the effect cannot last unless there is an increase in systemic venous return.

11.4.1 Venous return

Cardiac output relies upon recirculation of a more or less fixed volume of blood. The smaller the volume capacitance and the flow resistance of the vascular system, the faster the blood will recirculate.

Most of the capacitance of the system is accounted for by the venules and veins. Pooling of blood must be prevented: the less time blood spends in the veins, the sooner it will return to the heart. In exercising limbs, this is usually automatic, via the 'muscle-pump' effect. When limb muscles contract rhythmically, the deep veins are intermittently compressed and, provided their valves are competent, the blood is driven towards the heart. Once blood reaches the central veins, other mechanisms take over. One is the pumping effect produced by changes in differential pressure between abdomen and thorax during breathing. In inspiration, thoracic pressure falls, whereas abdominal pressure rises, compressing the abdominal veins and driving blood into the thorax. This effect is amplified by the greater

frequency and depth of breathing in exercise. The other major mechanisms
are vasomotor. The splanchnic and renal circulations, at rest, account for
50–55 per cent of cardiac output and hold approximately 25 per cent of
blood volume. We have already seen that, in maximal exercise, much of the
blood flow can be diverted to muscle. In addition, there is a marked generalized venoconstriction, which reduces the capacitance of the venous system
as a whole and that of the abdominal veins in particular. The initial increase
in venous return produced by these mechanisms can be regarded as a pump-
priming effect.

The other change which initiates and then sustains the increase in cardiac
output is the fall in total peripheral resistance, due to arteriolar dilatation in
working muscles. The resulting rise in blood flow through the muscles now
reappears as inflow to the veins and, thus, as a greater venous return. This
acts as a positive feedback which further increases cardiac output. The limit
to this process is set by the pumping capacity of the heart, that is, by heart
rate and stroke volume.

11.4.2 Heart rate

In a normal subject, heart rate rises approximately linearly with the severity
of exercise, towards a maximum of approximately 200 beats/min in a young
adult (Fig. 11.2). (Maximum heart rate declines with age to approximately
160 beats/min at 60 years.) The progressive rise is due at first to decreasing
vagal activity and then to a growing sympathetic drive.

The latter is probably mainly a direct nervous effect on the heart, though
circulating catecholamines can produce a substantial increase in the rate of
a denervated heart in exercise. The causes of the change in autonomic
activity are less clear. Like the generalized vasoconstriction and venoconstriction described earlier, it could be initiated by baroreceptor reflexes
if vasodilatation in working muscles led to a fall of arterial blood pressure.
However, the rise in heart rate closely parallels the peripheral vasoconstriction, with respect to both time and mechanisms (see p. 248). As the
heart rate increases, diastole shortens more than systole (thereby reducing
the time available for ventricular filling and for coronary blood flow).
Conduction within the heart is faster (shown by a shorter P-R interval in an
electrocardiogram) and there is some shortening of systole through an
increased velocity of contraction of cardiac muscle.

11.4.3 Stroke volume

In many cases, there must also be an increase in stroke volume during
exercise, since cardiac output often rises more than would be expected from
the increase in heart rate alone. The changes in stroke volume, though,
follow a different pattern from those in heart rate (Fig. 11.2). The most

marked rise occurs when a subject in the upright position undertakes moderate exercise. There is only a small further rise in maximal exercise, to approximately one and a half times the resting value. In the supine position, the stroke volume at rest is already larger than when upright and increases less when the subject exercises.

The mechanism of the increase is a source of much debate. A traditional explanation is based on Starling's 'Law of the Heart': greater filling by a higher venous pressure leads to a more forcible systole. However, there is no consistent relationship between right atrial pressure and stroke volume

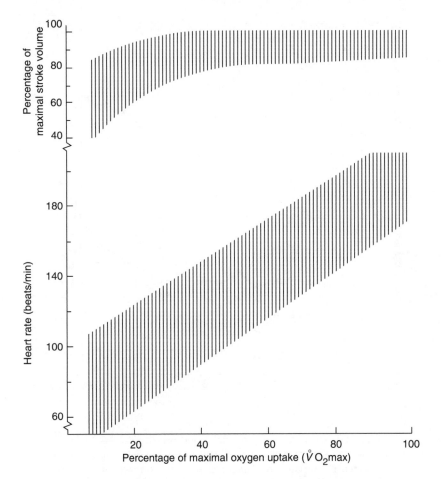

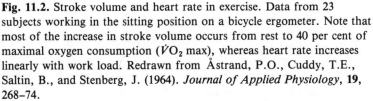

Fig. 11.2. Stroke volume and heart rate in exercise. Data from 23 subjects working in the sitting position on a bicycle ergometer. Note that most of the increase in stroke volume occurs from rest to 40 per cent of maximal oxygen consumption ($\dot{V}O_2$ max), whereas heart rate increases linearly with work load. Redrawn from Åstrand, P.O., Cuddy, T.E., Saltin, B., and Stenberg, J. (1964). *Journal of Applied Physiology*, **19**, 268–74.

and radiographic studies do not show any significant increase in end-diastolic volume in exercise. A more likely explanation is that there is a sympathetically produced increase in contractility, leading to more complete emptying in systole. Other factors may be the reduced peripheral resistance and more efficient filling. The non-linear increase in stroke volume and the effects of posture, suggest that it is not a closely controlled single effect but rather the result of several factors.

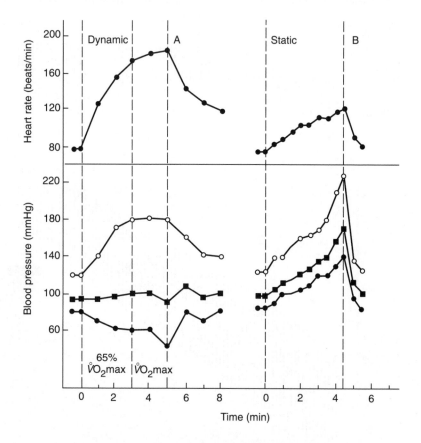

Fig. 11.3. Heart rate and arterial blood pressure (○——○, systolic; ●——●, diastolic; ■——■, mean) in (a) dynamic and (b) static (isometric) exercise. In dynamic exercise the subject ran on a treadmill at submaximal and maximal rates of oxygen consumption ($\mathring{V}O_2$ max). In static exercise he maintained a hand-grip at 30 per cent of maximal voluntary contraction (MVC). Note that, in dynamic exercise, the mean blood pressure rose little despite a large rise in heart rate; by implication, there must have been a large fall in peripheral resistance. Originally published in Lind, A.R. and McNicol, G.W. (1967). *Canadian Medical Association Journal*, **96**, 706–15.

11.4.4 Arterial blood pressure

Systolic pressure can rise to over 225 mmHg (30 kPa) in some kinds of exercise, though 190 mmHg (25 kPa) is a more typical limit. Diastolic pressure, on the other hand, shows only a small rise and in some subjects may fall slightly. Thus, pulse pressure may rise two- to three-fold (Fig. 11.3). The high systolic pressure results from ejection of the same (or larger) stroke volume in a shorter time, whereas the diastolic pressure reflects the close balance between increased cardiac output and reduced peripheral resistance. Note that values for blood pressure depend on how and where the pressure is measured. At high cardiac outputs, blood in the aorta has substantial kinetic as well as hydrostatic energy, so that pressure measured in line with flow is higher than that exerted laterally upon the vessel wall.

11.4.5 Coronary blood flow

Respiration in cardiac muscle is essentially aerobic. The heart is also very hardworking: even in a resting subject, its oxygen consumption is higher than that of any other organ, relative to its mass. This large oxygen supply is achieved by a combination of a generous blood flow (second only to the kidneys) and a high extraction of oxygen, that is, the venous blood is very desaturated. As in skeletal muscle (p. 238), blood flow in the coronary circulation is impeded by myocardial contraction. Flow ceases (or even reverses) in the wall of the left ventricle during isovolumetric contraction, rises transiently in the early part of ejection, then shows a sustained peak throughout diastole. Other chambers are less affected.

In dynamic exercise, cardiac work and oxygen consumption rise in proportion to heart rate. Diastole shortens, leaving less time for coronary flow. Nevertheless, because there is little scope for further venous desaturation, the extra oxygen has to come from increased blood flow, via vasodilatation. Hypoxia and adenosine are individually the most powerful coronary dilators, but there are probably synergistic effects between the various local factors.

11.5 Pulmonary oxygen uptake

Oxygen uptake in the lungs, like that in the muscles, is the product of blood flow (in this case, cardiac output) and arteriovenous difference of oxygen content (ΔavO_2). The 'arterialized' blood leaving the lungs is normally 95–97 per cent saturated with oxygen. Until a larger flow and/or more desaturated 'mixed venous' blood reaches the lungs, oxygen uptake cannot increase, whatever the increase in ventilation (except in so far as the thoracoabdominal pump hastens venous return).

11.5.1 **Flow and saturation of mixed venous blood**

At rest, there is a large venous flow from the renal and splanchnic circulations, which extract relatively little oxygen and a smaller flow from skeletal and heart muscle, of lower oxygen content. The oxygen saturation of the mixture reaching the lungs is therefore high (70–75 per cent) (Fig. 11.4). In exercise the splanchnic and renal flows decrease (and are probably more desaturated), whereas muscle flow increases greatly (and is even more desaturated). The mixed venous oxygen saturation falls towards that of exercising muscle and may reach as low as 20–25 per cent. Thus, each litre of cardiac output can accept up to three times more oxygen in the lungs than at rest, for example, 6–7 mmol (150 ml). Given a cardiac output four times that at rest, for example, 20 l/min, oxygen uptake can rise to 120–140 mmol (3 l)/min.

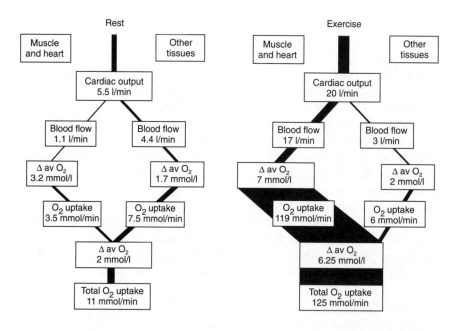

Fig. 11.4. Distribution of cardiac output and oxygen uptake at rest and in exercise. At rest, muscle and heart receive only 20 per cent of cardiac output but extract twice as much oxygen from each litre of blood as the rest of the body (i.e. arteriovenous difference of O_2 content ($\Delta av O_2$) is doubled). Thus, muscle and heart account for about 30 per cent of total oxygen uptake. In maximal exercise, the increase in cardiac output is directed entirely to muscle and heart, which now receive 85 per cent. Extraction of oxygen doubles, so that muscle and heart account for 95 per cent of total oxygen uptake.

11.5.2 Changes in pulmonary factors

There are three pulmonary factors that might limit pulmonary gas exchange and lead to an arterial oxygen saturation of less than 95–97 per cent: ventilation, diffusion, and matching of ventilation and perfusion. Ventilation does not appear to impose a limit, since healthy subjects are capable of levels of ventilation higher than the 100–150 l/min of maximal exercise. The pulmonary capillary bed is unlike that of resting muscle: there are few if any fully dormant capillaries. Instead, there is a marked regional variation in perfusion and blood volume, capillaries at the apices receiving little blood. When cardiac output increases in exercise, pulmonary blood pressure rises. The rise is small in absolute terms, 7–15 mmHg (1–2 kPa), but this is sufficient to produce a disproportionately large increase in apical blood flow and volume. This affects both diffusion and ventilation/perfusion.

The mean velocity of flow in individual capillaries approximately doubles, but since at rest blood reaches equilibrium with alveolar air before it is halfway through the capillary, there is still sufficient time for equilibration. The low PO_2 of the incoming blood also speeds diffusion. The larger volume of blood in apical capillaries increases the diffusing capacity approximately two-fold, though, like changes in stroke volume (see p. 240), this effect depends on posture and is not linearly related to intensity of exercise. In disorders where diffusing capacity is barely adequate at rest (pulmonary fibrosis, emphysema), there is no reserve and even light exercise results in a fall in arterial saturation.

The increase in apical blood flow which occurs during exercise is relatively greater than that in basal flow. Thus, blood flow becomes more evenly distributed within the lungs, and better matched to the distribution of ventilation.

Though ventilation, diffusion, and matching of ventilation and perfusion do not appear to limit pulmonary gas exchange in normal subjects, one or more of these may do so in highly athletic subjects. At oxygen consumptions greater than 120–140 mmol (3 l)/min (corresponding to cardiac outputs of 20–25 l/min), arterial PO_2 and saturation begin to fall. Since a modest increase in inspired oxygen concentration prevents the fall, it is likely that diffusion is the weak link—blood spends too short a time in the capillaries to reach equilibrium with alveolar air.

11.6 Static exercise

All movements begin with an isometric phase, during which there is contractile activity within muscle, but no overall shortening occurs. This continues until tension in the muscle rises to equal the applied load (whether this is the weight of the limb or some external load); at this point, movement begins. As the velocity of movement increases, tension in the muscle decreases, even though contractile activity continues. Eventually, as the planned movement nears completion, contractile activity ceases. The muscle relaxes and is then passively extended preparatory to repeating the movement; this cycle is typical in rhythmic exercise, such as walking and in the heart. The implications for blood flow in skeletal muscle (p. 238) and cardiac muscle (p. 243) have been noted already.

What happens if the cycle 'gets stuck' in the isometric phase because the load is immovable or if movement is very slow and prolonged because the load is almost overwhelming? At tensions up to 10–15 per cent of maximum, blood flow is unimpeded and tension can be maintained for long periods; this is presumably the situation in postural muscles. At greater tensions, there is progressive obstruction of blood flow until, at 50–70 per cent of maximum, blood flow ceases. There are consequences both for energy supply in muscle (see below) and for the rest of the cardiovascular system.

In any severe exercise, there are increases in sympathetic vasoconstrictor activity and in the frequency and force of cardiac contraction. In dynamic exercise these changes are balanced by metabolic vasodilatation in the working muscles, so that mean arterial pressure does not rise substantially (Fig. 11.3). In severe static exercise, however, resistance to flow through the working muscles rises, rather than falls. Thus, there are large rises in systolic, diastolic, and mean arterial pressures; via the baroreflex, the rise in heart rate is attenuated (Fig. 11.3). In terms of external work done by the heart (pressure × volume, plus kinetic energy), less work may be done than in dynamic exercise, because the volume pumped is less. On the other hand, the mechanical stresses on the heart and arterial system are greater and the energy consumption of the heart is higher for work done against an elevated pressure than for that done in pumping an increased volume.

11.7 Anaerobic energy sources

Anaerobic sources are called upon when the demand for energy exceeds the aerobic supply. This problem arises at the onset of any exercise, however mild, until the supply of oxygen catches up with demand—as it will in moderate dynamic exercise. However, in static exercise the oxygen supply may be cut off throughout; in severe dynamic exercise the demand for energy may exceed the maximum aerobic supply, because there is insufficient oxygen or inadequate mitochondrial capacity. In these latter cases, anaerobic energy must be used to replace or supplement the aerobic supply as long as exercise lasts. When the anaerobic reserves are exhausted, the exercise must cease or drop to a level which can be sustained aerobically (see p. 255).

11.7.1 'Oxygen deficit' and 'oxygen debt'

Energy 'borrowed' from anaerobic sources to finance the 'deficit' in aerobic energy must eventually be repaid, often 'with interest'. The energy to pay this total 'debt' (of 'deficit' plus 'interest') is 'earned' in the form of additional oxygen consumption after exercise.

The true 'oxygen debt' is small: the total oxygen content of the body is lower in exercise because the venous blood is more desaturated and some oxygen is extracted from myoglobin. In maximal exercise, such depletion of oxygen stores might supply 15–20 mmol (300–500 ml) of oxygen, equivalent to 7–9 kJ of aerobic energy. Most of the energy, though, is borrowed from two anaerobic sources: high-energy organic phosphates and anaerobic glycolysis.

11.7.2 High-energy phosphates

One of these, ATP, directly supplies energy for muscle contraction and is hydrolysed to ADP in the process (see p. 234). The other, creatine phosphate, is present in a concentration three to four times that of ATP in resting muscle and acts as a reserve from which ATP is regenerated. In heavy exercise, ATP concentration may fall by up to 30 per cent whereas creatine phosphate may fall by 80 per cent, thus supplying energy equivalent to consumption of 60–70 mmol (1.5 l) of oxygen or 30 kJ of aerobic energy. This source has the advantage of being instantly available and rapidly recharged after exercise (with a half-time of 20–30 s).

11.7.3 Anaerobic glycolysis

In the section on pathways of energy production (p. 234) it was noted that glycolysis can yield ATP in the absence of oxygen. The yield is small compared with aerobic metabolism (two or three ATP per 6-carbon unit of carbohydrate versus 38 or 39 ATP) and the relatively strong acid, lactic acid, accumulates. It plays a larger role in 'white' muscle (which has a high glycogenolytic capacity and is recruited in brief maximal efforts) than in 'red' (which has a higher aerobic capacity and is active over long periods). Though anaerobic glycolysis is most obvious when the demand for energy exceeds the aeriobic capacity, blood lactate concentration rises even when exercise intensity is only 50–60 per cent of maximal aerobic capacity.

In the short-term, the process is limited by the body's tolerance for lactic acid and the fall in pH it produces (see p. 255). Typically, blood lactate concentration rises from a resting value of 1–1.5 mmol/l to a peak of 10–15 mmol/l. When a large mass of muscle is active, 0.7–1.0 mmol of lactate can be produced, equivalent to 80–115 kJ of aerobic energy or 170–250 mmol (3.5–5.5 l) of oxygen consumed.

Lactate still in muscle at the end of exercise may revert to pyruvate and be oxidized through the citric acid cycle. However, the majority escapes into the blood. Some is oxidized by cardiac muscle, but the greater part (85 per cent) is synthesized into glycogen in the liver. This requires much more energy than the anaerobic glycolysis yielded, so that the final cost of repaying the 'debt' in terms of oxygen consumption is approximately double the original 'deficit'. Lactate production is slower in onset than depletion of creatine phosphate, taking 10–15 s to occur and recovery is very slow, taking 1 h or more. During recovery, the depleted carbohydrate stores are conserved by a shift towards oxidation of fat.

An example of the use of anaerobic energy sources is shown in Fig. 11.5. It is assumed that the subject reached a steady state after 8–10 min. The estimated oxygen 'deficit' is 117 mmol, but the 'debt' repaid is 244 mmol; this 'interest' reduced the net efficiency from 24.9 to 22.7 per cent. Components of 'interest' can be seen in the persistence of

(1) low pH, due to lactic acid;

(2) low Gas Exchange Ratio, R, due to oxidation of fat; and

(3) high rectal and skin temperature and heart rate.

In everyday life, it is likely that the fast depletion of oxygen and creatine phosphate can cover most brief or minor changes in physical activity and that anaerobic glycolysis is reserved for major efforts. In fact, it is possible to reach very high mean rates of work with very little lactate production or subjective exhaustion, by working in 10–15 s bursts separated by rest periods of 5–10 s, instead of working continuously at a lower load. Perhaps Aesop's hare was correct in his tactics!

11.8 Cardiorespiratory control

As we have seen, some of the adjustments occurring in exercise can be treated as simple cause and effect: increased extraction of oxygen from blood follows almost inevitably from increased oxygen uptake by the muscles. Other adjustments need at least a simple feedback control: stimulation of glycogenolysis by a fall in ATP. A further group could in theory be controlled by simple feedbacks but in practice obviously relies on more sophisticated controls: changes in heart rate, vasomotor activity, and breathing. Two aspects of the changes point to this conclusion: the values of blood pressure and blood gases found during exercise and the speed with which adjustments occur.

Heart rate, blood pressure, and sympathetic vasoconstrictor activity all rise during exercise—not what would be expected from operation of the baroreceptor reflex in a resting subject. Over a wide range of intensities of exercise, ventilation rises in close proportion to oxygen consumption and carbon dioxide production, but arterial PO_2 and PCO_2 show only small, erratic changes from resting values (approximately 7 mmHg (1 kPa)). Towards maximal intensity, ventilation rises faster than oxygen consumption and PCO_2 falls. Furthermore, adjustments begin before blood pressure

or blood gases have changed and reduce (or even reverse) the disturbance
before it has happened.

11.8.1 Changes at the beginning and end of exercise

Within the first 5–10 s of starting exercise, heart rate rises approximately
10–15 beats/min (Fig. 11.5); this is probably due more to decreased vagal
tone than to a sympathetic drive. There is often an even faster but more
erratic increase in ventilation of 5–20 l/min (Fig. 11.6). What happens next
depends very much on the severity of the exercise. In very light exercise,
there may be no further rise or even a slight fall in both variables. In
moderate exercise, there may be a brief hiatus before slower but larger and
more progressive rises towards steady levels. Most of the change occurs in
2–3 min, but there is a further gradual change up to 5–10 min. In heavy
exercise, the hiatus is not noticeable. In fact, the initial rapid change in
ventilation may not be seen, perhaps because the muscles of breathing are
compromised by the mechanical stress of the exercise.

At the end of exercise, the changes are more consistent: both heart rate
and ventilation fall sharply at first, then more slowly. The rapid changes at
the beginning and end are too quick to be explained by changes in the
composition or flow of venous blood and occur even when the circulation to
the exercising limbs is occluded. Chemoreceptor reflexes, if not suppressed,
are at least temporarily overridden: at the beginning, ventilation is rising
though PCO_2 is unchanged or falling. Heart rate and blood pressure both
rise. At the end, ventilation falls though PCO_2 is rising and heart rate and
blood pressure both fall: these relationships are not what would be expected
from the usual negative feedback reflexes.

11.8.2 Baroreceptor and chemoreceptor reflexes

Studies of baroreceptor reflex responses during exercise suggest that the
reflex is still active, but is reset to operate over a higher range of blood
pressures. At the same time, tonic vagal activity to the heart is decreased, so
that heart rate, cardiac output, and blood pressure rise. In moderate
dynamic exercise, this is sufficient to match the fall in peripheral resistance
due to metabolic vasodilatation in working muscles. In more severe dynamic
exercise, the blood pressure does not at first rise to the new target value, so
that there is, in addition, a reflex increase in sympathetic activity to the
heart and peripheral circulation. In static exercise, the increase in sympathetic activity may be driven by chemoreceptive reflexes from the ischaemic
muscles, rather than by the baroreceptor reflex.

There is some evidence that respiratory chemoreceptor reflexes are also
reset during exercise, though it is unclear which parameters change. It does
appear that there is a greater response to changes of PO_2 during exercise

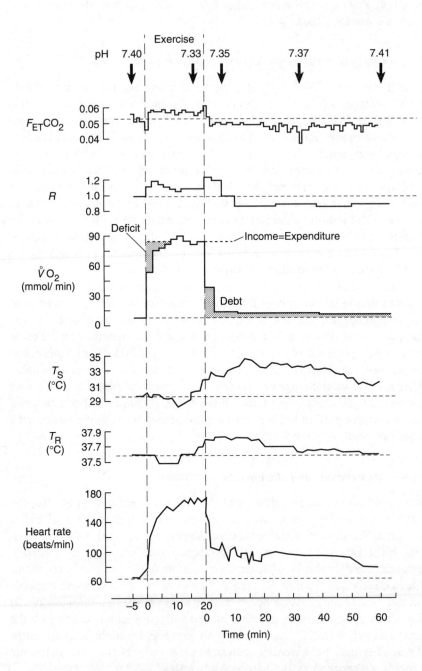

Fig. 11.5. Acid-base, metabolic, thermal, and cardiac changes during exercise and recovery. The subject worked in the sitting position on a bicycle ergometer at a load of 150 W. The broken horizontal lines represent mean pre-exercise values.

than there is at rest. In turn, this may indirectly influence response to carbon dioxide. In severe exercise, the rise in blood lactate provides an additional stimulus which causes ventilation to rise faster than oxygen consumption and carbon dioxide production.

11.8.3 Other evidence

In static exercise, both systolic and diastolic blood pressure rise progressively to very high values (Fig. 11.3). Despite this, heart rate also rises, though not as much as in heavy dynamic exercise: this suggests that baroreceptor reflexes may still partially counteract the imposed tachycardia. The more forcible the static muscular contraction, the larger and faster the rises in blood pressure and heart rate. Occlusion of the local circulation (which may already be impaired by the sustained contraction) tends to enhance the effect.

In dynamic exercise of small muscle groups (for example, an arm) ventilation, heart rate, and blood pressure are higher, for a given rate of oxygen uptake, than where large muscle groups are used. There is also evidence of a 'learning' effect, in that cardiorespiratory changes are smaller after training of the muscles. Where the central nervous 'command' is dissociated from the muscular force exerted (for example, by partial curarization), an increase in central command is accompanied by greater cardiorespiratory changes. Passive and, in particular, electrically stimulated limb movements have also been shown to increase breathing, heart rate, and blood pressure. Selective blockade, however, suggests that C-fibres (rather than the larger proprioceptive afferents) are principally responsible once exercise is in progress. The stimuli may then be chemical changes in the muscles.

Note: (1) During exercise and much of recovery, arterial blood pH was lower than would be expected from end-tidal carbon dioxide concentration ($F_{ET}CO_2$), implying a non-respiratory acidosis.

(2) During exercise and early recovery, the gas exchange ratio (R) was above unity, implying that more carbon dioxide was being eliminated by ventilation than was being produced by tissue respiration.

(3) Of the oxygen debt, 35 per cent was repaid within the first 3 min of recovery and 48 per cent (equivalent to the initial deficit) in 11 min; the remaining debt was repaid very slowly.

(4) Skin temperature (T_S) changed after rectal temperature (T_R); the initial fall in T_R may be due to cooler venous blood from the legs; most of the surplus heat was eliminated during recovery, not exercise.

(5) Heart rate rose and fell rapidly at beginning and end of exercise; the rise immediately before exercise was probably due to anticipation, and the slow decline during recovery may reflect skin blood flow (see (4), above).

11.8.4 Conclusions

There is probably some central cardiorespiratory activation at the beginning of exercise which is not closely related to the severity of exercise but is linked to initiation of movement. This accounts for the initial rise in ventilation seen in the first few seconds of Fig. 11.6. Increased ventilation cannot increase oxygen uptake at this stage, but may pre-empt a lactic acidosis and increase venous return. It is later reinforced or attenuated according to the central 'command' the exercise demands and also perhaps by information from chemosensitive nerves in muscle. These account for a secondary rise during the first minute of Fig. 11.6. This further boost

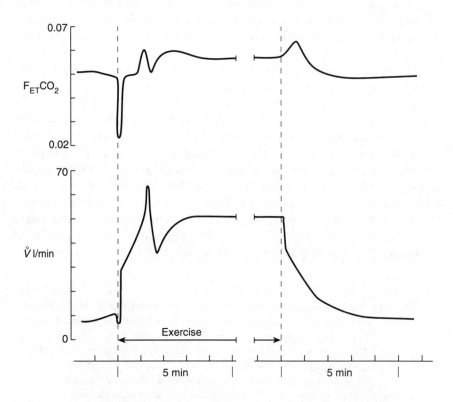

Fig. 11.6. Respiratory changes at the beginning and end of exercise. These are details from the experiment shown in Fig. 11.5. Note:
(1) The brief fall in end-tidal carbon dioxide concentration $F_{ET}CO_2$ at the beginning of exercise may be an artefact, but ventilation ($\mathring{V}_I$) clearly rises before $F_{ET}CO_2$.
(2) The initial peak of $\mathring{V}_I$ at 1–1.5 min is not sustained; it is succeeded at 2–3 min by a slower rise which follows the rise in $F_{ET}CO_2$.
(3) $\mathring{V}_I$ falls rapidly during the first 0.5 min of recovery, despite the rise in $F_{ET}CO_2$ which results.

appears to have run a little ahead of the need for gas exchange: the end tidal concentration of carbon dioxide and the ventilation then show a temporary fall before stabilizing at the levels which continue to the end of exercise. Since, in dynamic exercise, blood pressure appears quite well controlled, though at a higher level, it is likely that baroreceptor reflexes persist but are superimposed on a higher basal sympathetic activity. The role of the respiratory chemoreceptors may be even simpler, namely that they continue to function as at rest (though perhaps with an enhanced response to hypoxia). Since they lie in the arterial circulation, they do not detect the load of carbon dioxide reaching the lungs or the level of ventilation, but rather any failure of ventilation to eliminate carbon dioxide. Given that breathing has been elevated by other factors to an approximately adequate level before the full flow of deoxygenated carbon dioxide-laden blood arrives at the lungs, only minor corrections will be needed to reach a new steady state.

The control of breathing in exercise is a source of much debate. There are many interpretations more elaborate than the one above, each with some experimental evidence in its favour.

11.9 Temperature, fluid, and acid–base disturbances

11.9.1 Efficiency of exercise

Of the energy released when carbohydrate or fat is oxidized to carbon dioxide and water, the greater part appears as heat. Generation of ATP by oxidative phosphorylation has an efficiency of approximately 50 per cent and anaerobic glycolysis is less efficient (even when the lactate is recycled; see p. 247). Further losses of energy occur as heat when ATP is used in muscle contraction. Overall, only approximately 25 per cent of the original chemical energy of carbohydrates or fat can be realized as useful mechanical work.

In exercise on a bicycle ergometer, it is relatively easy to estimate the total work done, but in running on the flat or in swimming, most of the work lies in acceleration and deceleration of the limbs and in overcoming viscosity. The apparent efficiency of exercise depends very much on the allowances made for 'invisible' work and for basal energy consumption. Marginal (or 'net') efficiency calculated from the difference in energy expenditure between running on the flat and running uphill is obviously higher than the gross efficiency calculated from total energy expenditure. By definition, the efficiency of static (isometric) exercise is nil, since the load is not moved. The energy cost of 'negative' or 'eccentric' work (where an active muscle is stretched by a load) is far less than in 'positive' work. Mathematically inclined readers may calculate whether the resulting efficiency is large or negative (or both!).

11.9.2 **Temperature regulation**

Clearly, the extra heat produced by exercise must be disposed of. In a short sprint this is no problem, because the quantity of heat is small and some of it is associated with the repayment of oxygen debt during recovery. At the beginning of exercise, there may even be a small fall of core temperature as venous return from the (initially) cooler limbs increases. This may lead to a fall in skin temperature.

In moderate exercise of longer duration, even in hot environments (for example, 35°C), the rise in core temperature is only approximately 1°C. Most of the extra heat is generated outside the body core and a substantial proportion may be eliminated directly from the exercising limbs. Also, sweating begins at a lower core temperature during exercise than at rest. Of course, skin blood flow increases very greatly at the higher environmental temperatures, but cardiac output rises to supply the flow. There is also an increase in heat loss by evaporation from the respiratory tract.

In sustained heavy exercise in a hot environment, the needs of exercise and thermoregulation conflict. Cardiac output is already maximal and skin blood flow can rise only at the cost of some other tissue. Visceral vaso-constriction intensifies to the verge of hepatic failure through ischaemia and rising temperature. Skin blood flow rises, but not enough, so that core temperature rises progressively. Stroke volume decreases as a result of pooling of blood in cutaneous veins and a reduction in plasma volume (see below). Eventually, cardiac output, arterial blood pressure, and oxygen uptake fall. Sometimes, this effect is seen soon after exercise stops: cuta-neous blood flow is rising but leg movements have ceased and venous pooling occurs—the subject may even faint.

11.9.3 **Plasma volume; sweating**

In heavy exercise, as much as 15 per cent of plasma volume shifts into the interstitial space of muscle. This is due to increased hydrostatic pressure within the vasodilated capillaries and to accumulation of osmotically active substances in the interstitium. Provided that cardiac output is not affected, this haemoconcentration may slightly increase delivery of oxygen to the working muscles.

More serious, in exercise of long duration, is the outright loss of water and sodium ions in sweat. In moderate exercise at an ambient temperature of 15°C, the sweat rate is approximately 0.2–0.3 l/h, but at 35°C can reach 1.5 l/h. Loss of K^+ to the interstitium may also cause weakness.

11.9.4. **Acid–base balance**

Carbonic acid is potentially a major threat to acid–base balance since in heavy exercise carbon dioxide production can reach 100 mmol/min. Retention of one minute's production would approximately double the hydrogen ion concentraiton in blood (pH would drop 0.3 units). Normally, of course, carbon dioxide is eliminated as fast as it is produced (or even faster at the beginning of exercise if there is an anticipatory increase of ventilation). Buffering of this larger quantity in venous blood is automatic under aerobic conditions, since haemoglobin is more desaturated.

In practice, the major threat arises from lactic acid produced in the course of anaerobic glycolysis (see p. 247). When a subject exercises to exhaustion in 1–3 min and employs a large mass of muscle, 0.7–1.0 mol of lactate is formed. During such a short period, there is little time for lactate to leave the muscle and intramuscular pH falls from a resting value of approximately 7.0 to 6.4–6.6 at exhaustion. In muscle venous blood, pH may fall to 7.0 or below: this is in part a reflection of the high PCO_2, due to both aerobic production and buffering of lactate by bicarbonate. In arterial blood (where PCO_2 is lower), the pH reaches a minimum of 7.1–7.2 some 5–10 min after the end of exercise. In exercise to exhaustion over a longer time course, arterial pH may fall even further, presumably because there is more time for lactate to escape from the muscles (though some may then be disposed of metabolically).

The fall in arterial pH stimulates breathing, so that total ventilation increases out of proportion to oxygen consumption and carbon dioxide production by the tissues. The gas exchange ratio (R) rises far above unity as carbon dioxide elimination increases and arterial PCO_2 falls below the resting value. This respiratory compensation is, of course, a temporary expedient: the acid–base disturbance will be fully corrected only when the lactate has been removed during the lengthy recovery from exercise (Fig. 11.5). As the lactate is removed, carbon dioxide is retained; this, together with a shift towards oxidation of fat, reduces R below its preexercise level.

11.10 Endurance and training

11.10.1 Endurance

As one might expect, there is an inverse relationship between intensity and duration of exercise. Maximal efforts, whether static or brief dynamic, are essentially anaerobic. The total force exerted will depend on the muscle mass and its composition: weightlifters and sprinters, for example, have a higher than average proportion of 'white' fibres in their leg muscles. Such an effort can be maintained for only a few seconds—perhaps barely long enough for anaerobic glycolysis to occur. A half-maximal isometric contraction can be sustained for 1–2 min and a 15 per cent contraction almost indefinitely (see p. 246).

A similar pattern applies to dynamic exercise. There is a limited quantity of anaerobic energy available (100–150 kJ, see p. 247) which will last approximately 20–30 s at full power: a sprinter runs as fast for 200 m as for 100 m, but is slower over 400 m. Alternatively, the same quantity of energy can be spread over a longer period to supplement, rather than to replace, the aerobic supply. Over 1000 m (2.5 min), roughly half the energy used is anaerobic; the remainder comes from oxidative phosphorylation, which by now has reached its maximum rate. Over 20 km (1 h), the anaerobic energy is spread so thinly that its contribution is negligible. The runner is reduced to an aerobic plateau which is approximately only 50 per cent of the maximal aerobic capacity in an untrained subject (see p. 247); a highly trained athletic subject might achieve 80 per cent.

Over longer periods of several hours, there is a further slow decline in power. One factor in this is depletion of glycogen stores: those in muscle reach very low levels in one hour of heavy exercise and the falling blood glucose concentration suggests that liver glycogen is depleted too. The falling respiratory quotient and rising oxygen consumption confirm the growing dependence on fat. Diet has a marked effect on endurance over these longer periods. In particular, if glycogen stores have been previously emptied by exhaustion, a carbohydrate-rich diet can raise muscle glycogen to twice the normal concentration and can correspondingly double the endurance for sustained heavy work.

Disturbances of fluid and electrolyte balance and the need for thermoregulation will also, of course, limit endurance, particularly in adverse environments (see p. 254).

11.10.2 Local changes

To some extent, the effects of training are specific because a skilled movement is perfected. Irrelevant movement is decreased and energy is expended to better effect. In particular, in sustained exercise, there is less recruitment of 'white' muscle and greater reliance on the more enduring 'red' muscles. Even when the skill has been learned, though, major changes continue to occur in the muscles.

An obvious change is that of muscle mass, as in a 'professional strongman'. This is misleading: such gross hypertrophy is a specialized adaptation to static exercise, though it may also be seen, to a lesser extent, in the leg muscles of a sprinter. The larger muscles can exert larger forces, but not for long. Without corresponding cardiovascular adaptation, dynamic endurance is not increased. It may even be reduced because blood flow is inadequate for the greater mass of tissue. Of course, this hardly matters during a maximal isometric contraction, since the blood flow ceases (see p. 238). To be effective, training for anaerobic power must place demands on anaerobic energy sources. The subject should exercise to exhaustion as rapidly as possible (for example, in 1 min) as often as possible (for example, every 5 min); this is unpleasant.

At the other extreme, middle- and long-distance runners show relatively modest changes in size and force of the leg muscles, but possess very great endurance. In addition to some increase in the size of the fibres, a number of biochemical and local cardiovascular changes occur in dynamically trained muscles. In general, these changes result in a greater capacity to produce energy aerobically.

The biochemical pattern varies with the type of muscle fibre. 'White' muscle has a high myosin ATPase activity and glycogenolytic capacity, but a low hexokinase activity and aerobic capacity. 'Red' fibres show species variation, but tend to the opposite. In 'endurance' training (which for this purpose means repeated bursts of 3–5 min or longer), the main changes are seen in the 'red' fibres. Mitochondrial density and the concentrations of hexokinase, citric acid cycle enzymes, cytochromes, and myoglobin increase, whereas glycogen phosphorylase may decrease (see p. 235). Overall, there is increased storage of glycogen and triglyceride and greater use of free fatty acids as a substrate. Glycogen stores are depleted less rapidly and less lactate is produced at a given intensity of exercise. On the other hand, higher lactate concentrations (of 20 mmol/l or more) can be tolerated. Thus, a greater continuous intensity of exercise can be sustained over longer periods.

An increased aerobic capacity implies an increased supply of oxygen. Part of this results from greater desaturation of muscle venous blood in trained subjects, but the mechanism is not quite clear. There is probably some increase in total capillary density (to be distinguished from opening existing but dormant capillaries, see p. 237). The greater mitochondrial density may also enhance diffusion by lowering intramuscular PO_2. There is evidence of a larger shift of the oxyhaemoglobin dissociation curve under working conditions, associated with an increased concentration of 2,3-diphosphoglycerate in red cells; however, this shift is not apparent under standard conditions *in vitro*. Following training, there is a greater maximal blood flow to muscle, related in part to the greater muscle mass. On the other hand, the blood flow at a given work load is not higher in the trained subject. It may even be lower, because each volume of blood unloads more oxygen.

11.10.3 General changes

The changes described above (apart from that in the oxyhaemoglobin dissociation curve) are specific to the trained muscles; more general cardiovascular changes may also occur. Two or three months of endurance training, involving a large proportion of total muscle mass and near-maximal rates of oxygen consumption, increases both maximal cardiac output and oxygen uptake (see Fig. 11.7a). Cardiac output at a given work load is not higher and may be lower. The training should be heavy enough to elicit

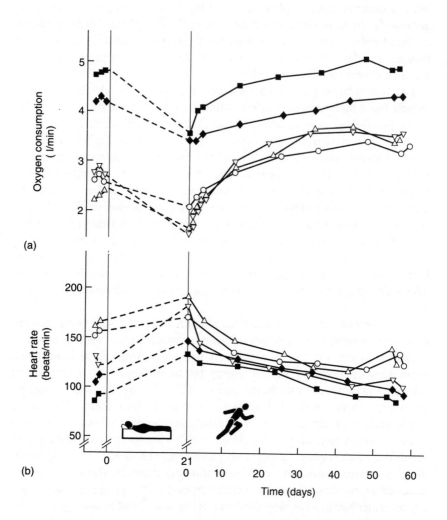

Fig. 11.7. Effects of bed-rest and training on (a) oxygen uptake during
maximal treadmill exercise and (b) heart rate during submaximal exercise
(an oxygen consumption of 1.5 litres·min^{-1}). Before the study, three
subjects ($\bigcirc$, $\triangle$, $\triangledown$) were healthy but athletically inactive; the other two
($\blacksquare$, $\blacklozenge$) were highly active. The effects of three weeks bed-rest followed
by two months of strenuous training were qualitatively similar in all
subjects, though the changes were relatively greater in the non-athletic.
Two subjects ($\triangle$, $\triangledown$) fainted when first exercised after bed-rest. Redrawn
from Saltin, B., Blomqvist, G., Mitchell, J.H., Johnson, R.L. Jr.,
Wildenthal, K., and Chapman, C.B. (1968). Response to exercise after
bed-rest and after training. A longitudinal study of adaptive changes in
oxygen transport and body composition. *Circulation*, **38**, No. 5,
Supplement No. VII, by permission of the American Heart Association Inc.

near-maximal heart rate and oxygen consumption for a few minutes, but need not be so heavy or prolonged that the subject is exhausted. Submaximal exercise or training of smaller muscle masses has less effect, presumably because total cardiac output is not a limiting factor. Longer term training is associated with enlargement of the heart; in endurance exercise the change is in end-diastolic volume, but in static exercise the change is in ventricular wall thickness, reflecting the high arterial pressures that occur (see p. 246 and Fig. 11.3).

Maximal heart rate does not change with training. However, a characteristic effect of training is a lower resting heart rate, which implies a larger stroke volume. As a result, the trained subject can achieve a given work load and cardiac output at a lower heart rate (see Fig. 11.7b). There is also a proportionate reduction in splanchnic and renal vasoconstriction. Quite light training can lower heart rate: in a group of habitually sedentary women, 5 min of rope skipping each day for a month reduced mean heart rate during the exercise from 168 to 145 beats/min. Since the maximal heart rate is unchanged, there is scope for a greater maximal cardiac output and work load. The mechanism of the lower resting heart rate is uncertain: possibly there is a higher vagal tone. It may, however, be just one manifestation of a wider change in autonomic, particularly sympathetic, activity.

In heavy exercise of small untrained muscle groups (for example, the arms), heart rate and ventilation are higher in relation to work load and oxygen consumption than when large muscle groups are used (see p. 251). After training of these muscles, the rises in ventilation, heart rate, and blood pressure are smaller and there is less splanchnic vasoconstriction. These changes do not 'carry over' to exercise in general, unlike the changes that follow maximal training of large muscle masses.

If training ceases, the heart rate reverts towards its pre-training level in the course of a few weeks (see Fig. 11.7). Bed-rest produces a corresponding temporary rise of heart rate, at rest and in exercise. The temporary nature of these changes and their specificity to particular muscle groups, do not suggest that they are due to permanent structural modifications of the heart or vascular system. Rather, they may represent a 'learning' process which modifies the autonomic and respiratory responses to exercise.

There is often some increase in blood volume and total red cell mass (though not in haematocrit or haemoglobin concentration). Tolerance of dehydration and the capacity to sweat may be greater with long endurance training. There are no changes in lung volumes or in ventilation or diffusing capacity except those that follow from increased maximal cardiac output and oxygen uptake.

11.10.4 Clinical aspects

For a patient with cardiorespiratory disorder, everyday tasks may constitute maximal exercise. The burden can be eased by avoiding or modifying some activities. For example, exercise involving small muscle groups or sustained contractions can put greater stress upon the heart than dynamic exercise of large muscle groups (see pp. 243 and 251 and Fig. 11.3). It may also be less exhausting to work hard intermittently than to work continuously at a lower load (see p. 248).

On the other hand, regular physical activity plays an important role in both prevention and treatment of myocardial ischaemia. The benefits may arise in several ways: from a reduction in heart rate (thereby increasing the time for coronary blood flow, see p. 243), from increased calibre of coronary blood vessels, and from changes in blood lipids.

Heart rate is a useful simple criterion of the stress imposed by dynamic exercise. Very approximately, a heart rate 30 beats/min below the expected maximum (see p. 240) corresponds to 70 per cent maximal oxygen consumption. This is usually a safe work load for a few minutes, though a subject with respiratory (rather than cardiovascular) disorder may become intolerably breathless before reaching this level. In particular, in disorders that increase the work of breathing (for example, airways obstruction), the effort required to breathe and the consequent oxygen consumption by the ventilatory muscles can severely limit exercise capacity. In any case, it is wise to raise the load in steps and to stop if any distress or cardiac irregularity appears. Particular care is needed where the subject has recently been confined to bed for *any* reason. In five healthy subjects, maximal stroke volume and cardiac output decreased by 5–49 per cent during 3 weeks of bed-rest, and two of the subjects fainted upon maximal exercise (see Fig. 11.7 and Chapter 9).

11.11 Work and play

Daily energy expenditure may range from 5 MJ per 24 h (equivalent to a mean power of 60 W) for a small female student in a hot climate, to 25 MJ (300 W) for a large Scandinavian lumberjack in winter. More typical would be 8–10 MJ (90–115 W) for women and 10–12 MJ (115–140 W) for men. Within the day there are even wider variations in power consumption. Whereas the student's rate could barely fall any lower (perhaps 50 W, in sleep), the lumberjack skiing to work or wielding his axe may reach 1.3 kW. Suppose he sleeps 8 h (3 MJ) and eats, drinks, and plays cards for 8 h (5 MJ). His mean power consumption during the 8 h work shift will be only 590 W, that is, he spends more than half the shift leaning on his axe, getting his breath back. As he tires or ages, he will reduce his mean work rate by taking longer rest periods (or by promotion to foreman). Running steadily at 8 km/h (5 mph) uses energy as fast as the lumberjack's mean rate, but is less exhausting because the runner is using only 50–60 per cent of maximal aerobic capacity and little lactate is formed (see p. 248). This illustrates two important points: that the duration of exercise is at least as significant as its intensity in determining the total work done and that some ways of working are more exhausting than others.

Similar principles apply to play, with the difference that the player may have more latitude in adjusting mean power consumption. For example, in a hard game of squash, the rate can be as high as 1.2 kW, but in a desultory game with frequent pauses, it will be much lower. In some team games (for example, football), the mean rate may be quite low, many players using more energy standing shivering than in chasing the ball. On the other hand, the total energy expenditure of a novice playing a full round of golf may be high, due to surplus strokes and searching for lost balls.

Apparently similar sports can make different demands. Cross-country skiing requires a very large aerobic capacity: one skier had a maximal oxygen uptake of 7.4l/min (equivalent to 2.47 kW). Downhill skiers do not have such large aerobic capacities, but show great isometric strength in the extensor muscles of their legs. Walking is more economical than slow running (or jogging) but the energy cost rises sharply with speed, for example, from 150 J/m at 4 km/h (2.5 mph) to over 300 J/m at 8 km/h (5 mph). The cost of running for the same 75 kg subject was reasonably constant at 300 J/min over a range 4–14 km/h (2.5–8.5 mph). Moral: if you get tired running, don't slow to a jog but walk. On the other hand, if you are trying to slim, jogging for long distances is a good way of burning off fat, whereas sprinting would use mainly carbohydrate (see p. 235).

In most sports, the fat subject carries a built-in weight penalty; in swimming, this is not so. There are even advantages, in that less energy is used to keep the swimmer afloat and (in British coastal waters) at the right working temperature (see Chapter 6). This may be why women are somewhat more efficient swimmers than men. Style and technique make large differences to efficiency. Freestyle (crawl) is more efficient than breaststroke and butterfly is particularly inefficient. Whereas the skilled runner or cyclist is not much more efficient than the untrained subject, there are large differences between swimmers. In freestyle the leg stroke is almost irrelevant, unless flippers are worn. With arms alone, the speed is almost as high and the efficiency is higher; the main effect of the leg stroke is to keep the body horizontal. Correspondingly, trained swimmers have a high proportion of 'red' fibres in the shoulder muscles but not in their thighs.

In conclusion, if you choose a sport as a means of keeping fit, decide what you want to achieve first. On the other hand, if you just want to enjoy it, take your pick.

Further reading

American Physiological Society Symposium (1984). Regulation in physiological systems during exercise in trained and untrained subjects. *Federation Proceedings*, **44**, 2259–2300.

American Physiological Society Symposium (1985). Anaerobiosis, lactate, and gas exchange during exercise I and II. *Federation Proceedings*, **45**, 2904–57.

Åstrand, P.-O. and Rodahl, K. (1987). *Textbook of work physiology*, 3rd edn. McGraw-Hill, New York.

Booth, F.W. and Thomason, D.B. (1991). Molecular and cellular adaptation of muscle in response to exercise: perspectives of various models. *Physiological Reviews*, **71**, 541–85.

Cotes, J.E. (1979). *Lung function: assessment and application in medicine*, 4th edn, Blackwell, Oxford. Chapter 12: Assessment of respiratory control and the physiological response to exercise.

Cunningham, D.J.C. (1987). Studies on arterial chemoreceptors in man. *Journal of Physiology*, **384**, 1–26.

Rowell, L.B. and O'Leary, D.S. (1990). Reflex control of the circulation during exercise: chemoreflexes and mechanoreflexes. *Journal of Applied Physiology*, **69**, 407–18.

12

Injury (shock)

12.1 Introduction

'Between the ages of 1 and 29, accidents are by far the most common cause of death.'

Royal Society for the Prevention of Accidents/
National Association of Health Authorities (1990)

Accidental injury is the commonest reason for attendance at a hospital casualty department in Western Europe. In the United Kingdom approximately 4 million people are sufficiently injured to attend hospital each year. Of these, 400 000 are admitted and approximately 14 000 die. Half of these deaths are a result of road traffic accidents, which is the single largest cause of death in males up to 40 years old. In this age group, the fatal injuries are major or multiple. But in the elderly (those aged over 65 years) much less severe injuries, such as a fractured neck or femur, have a 1-year mortality rate of 50 per cent. Perhaps the greatest burden that accidents impose on society is the expense of prolonged in-patient treatment and rehabilitation, together with the loss of working time.

The responses of the body to injury can be most conveniently divided into local (that is, responses in the injured tissues) and general (the response elicited in the rest of the body by the local response). The latter can be referred to as 'shock' and it is in this context that the term has been used in this chapter. Many forms of shock can be distinguished, each of which describes the pattern of responses to a particular injury or insult, for example, traumatic shock (response to trauma), haemorrhagic shock (response to haemorrhage), septic or endotoxic shock (response to infection), and cardiogenic shock (response to heart failure). Attempts to define shock on the basis of a reduced cardiac output (or, more accurately, reduced tissue perfusion) may have more scientific appeal but they are not very satisfactory as they presume knowledge of what is an adequate cardiac output at all stages of the response to injury. Furthermore, in septic shock, cardiac output and tissue perfusion may actually be raised. Irreversible shock, which refers to the terminal phase of the response preceding death, is characterized by a reduced cardiac output and failure of tissue perfusion (see later).

This chapter illustrates the challenge that injury provides to homoeostatic reflexes and, hopefully, may stimulate interest in this neglected area of study.

12.2 The local response to injury

When a tissue suffers direct injury, it soon shows the four classic signs of inflammation described in the first century AD by Celsus. They are redness (or flare), swelling, an increase in tissue temperature (heat), and pain. These may be followed by a fifth sign, loss of function, added by Virchow in the mid-nineteenth century. The first three of these signs can be directly attributed to changes in the microcirculation (venules, capillaries, and arterioles) in the injured tissue. The redness is due to vasodilatation of arterioles, heat to increased blood flow, and swelling to an increase in the extravascular fluid content of the injured tissues (oedema). This post-traumatic oedema is a result of an increase in microvascular permeability and is therefore an exudate. Of course, if blood vessels are directly damaged and ruptured, whole blood will also be lost at the site of the injury, either escaping to the outside or being retained in the tissue as a bruise or haematoma.

Although discussion of the local response to injury will be limited to inflammation, it should not be forgotten that fractures and direct damage to underlying tissues such as muscle and deeper organs (for example, liver and brain) can occur as part of a localized response to injury.

12.2.1 Vascular changes in inflammation

The increase in microvascular permeability may result from direct damage to the endothelium (this can affect all vessels in the microcirculation) or be secondary to the release of an intermediary or mediators at the site of injury, such as histamine, 5-hydroxytryptamine, bradykinin, and arachidonic acid metabolites (for example, leukotrienes).

Histamine, released from mast cells in the injured tissue, has two main effects on the microcirculation. It causes arteriolar dilatation (hence, the redness or flare of the response) and contraction of the endothelial cells in the non-muscular venules. When they contract, the endothelial cells pull away from each other creating 'leaks' in the vessel walls.

What happens after injury will depend on its severity. Following a very minor injury or at the edge of a more severe injury or after the injection of histamine into the skin, there is an immediate increase in venular permeability. This reaction lasts only 15 min. If the injury is more severe, this early phase is followed by a second, delayed increase in venular and/or capillary permeability which may be prolonged and therefore of greater significance. The mediator of this delayed phase has not yet been identified. After a severe injury, such as a major burn, the immediate and delayed phases become indistinguishable and there is rapid and sustained loss of fluid from all vessels in the microcirculation.

An important component of inflammation involves the interaction between leukocytes (for example, neutrophils) and vascular endothelial cells. The leukocytes adhere to the endothelial cells following the expression of surface adhesion molecules such as the integrins and selectins. Adherent leukocytes which have been activated by inflammatory mediators can change endothelial barrier function in a number of ways, for example, by the release of toxic oxygen products and proteases. The extent of change can vary from an increase in permeability (such that macromolecules escape) to separation of the endothelial cells from the basement membrane, allowing the passage of blood cells into the interstitium.

12.2.2 Modification of the local response

Fluid loss is influenced by a number of factors. Some of these are included in Starling's equation, as modified by Landis and Pappenheimer, which describes the movement of fluid across the microvascular endothelium as a balance between a number of forces:

$$FM = K(P_c - \pi_{PL} - P_{IF} + \pi_{IF})$$

where FM is fluid movement, K is the capillary filtration coefficient (a measure of microvascular permeability and of the surface area available for exchange), P_c is capillary pressure, π_{PL} is plasma protein osmotic pressure, P_{IF} is interstitial fluid pressure (tissue pressure), and π_{IF} is protein osmotic pressure in interstitial fluid immediately outside vessels.

It is difficult to decide what effect the capillary filtration coefficient and osmotic forces will have when selective permeability has been reduced or lost after injury. However, accumulation of protein-rich exudate in the damaged tissue may be a factor tending to move and retain fluid within the extravascular space. The picture is a little clearer when we consider the hydrostatic pressures. If capillary hydrostatic pressure is increased, fluid movement out of the circulation will increase. Conversely, with a low capillary pressure, leakage may not occur. Thus, the true extent of tissue injury may be masked in accident victims with severely reduced blood pressure, in whom oedema only becomes obvious when they are resuscitated and blood pressure rises.

A rise in tissue hydrostatic pressure will tend to limit post-traumatic fluid loss from damaged vessels. This mechanism provides a natural limitation to the amount of swelling that occurs after injury and can be assisted by the application of external strapping. The rise in tissue pressure will largely depend on the laxity or compliance of the tissues; for example, compare the marked swelling which occurs around the injured eye, where the tissues are lax, with that over the injured shin, where the tissues are tightly bound together. Oedema will also be influenced by the ability of the lymph vessels to carry away the extra tissue fluid and return it to the circulation through the thoracic duct.

Other factors that can modify the amount of fluid lost after injury include tissue temperature, age, and the presence of pre-existing disease. A reduction in temperature of the injured tissue, occurring as the result either of an overall fall in body temperature (hypothermia) or the local application of cold, will reduce oedema formation. The permeability of the microcirculation of the newborn and young infant is not increased by factors such as histamine. However, post-traumatic fluid loss is greater in the very young perhaps because of the greater laxity of the tissues at that age. A disease such as diabetes mellitus modifies the local response to injury; the predisposition of diabetics to infection is a result of their impaired ability to mount an inflammatory response.

Pharmacological agents can also limit the acute inflammatory response. These include antagonists of the classical permeability factors (for example, antihistamines), steroidal agents such as the glucocorticoids which can block the release of cytokines from macrophages, and non-steroidal anti-inflammatory agents which modify the release of arachidonic acid metabolites. Cytokines such as tumour necrosis factor or cachectin, interleukin-1 or endogenous pyrogen, and interleukin-6 are a family which mediate local and systemic responses characteristic of trauma and infection. They may provide the link between the local and general responses.

12.2.3 Cellular phase of inflammation

Although the most obvious external sign of inflammation is swelling, of more importance for defence against the effects of local tissue injury is the accumulation of leukocytes at the site of injury. As described above, the circulating leukocytes first adhere to the blood vessel walls and then migrate across the venular walls between endothelial cells. Once in the injured tissues, the leukocytes phagocytize cellular debris and any invading bacteria.

12.3 The cause of the general response to injury (initiating factors)

What feature or features of the local response are responsible for triggering the general response in the rest of the body? There are three candidates:

(1) fluid loss from the circulation;

(2) release of toxic factors from the injured tissues; and

(3) afferent nervous impulses from the site of injury.

12.3.1 Fluid loss from the circulation

The volume of fluid lost after a large burn or rupture of a major vessel is obviously considerable. What is not always appreciated is the magnitude of the loss frequently associated with less severe injuries (Table 12.1). For example, even after a closed fracture of the thigh bone, the loss can be as high as 2 l, which is a large amount when one recalls that the total blood volume of a 70 kg man is approximately 5 l.

Table 12.1. Fluid loss after injury in the adult human

Injury	Fluid loss (litres)
Fracture–dislocation, ankle	0.25–0.5
Closed fracture, lower leg	0.5 –1.0
Closed fracture, thigh	0.5 –2.0
Open (compound) fracture, thigh	1.0 –3.0
Multiple rib fractures	1.0 –2.0

Fluid loss from the circulation is probably the most important cause of the general response to injury. Consequently, a major component of this response involves compensating for this fluid loss in an attempt to maintain tissue blood supply; this will be discussed later.

12.3.2 Toxic factors

The search for toxic factors was largely stimulated by Cannon and Bayliss, who considered that the fluid loss after injury was insufficient to account for the circulatory failure frequently seen in battle casualties during the First World War. If they had measured intravascular volumes, as others did during the Second World War, they would have appreciated the true magnitude of the loss. The concept of a toxic factor being generated in the injured tissues and liberated into the circulation to 'poison' the rest of the body is very plausible. Consequently, many factors have been suggested, ranging from simple ions (for example, K^+), hormones (noradrenalin), inflammatory mediators (histamine, cytokines), and metabolites (lactate) to factors extracted from injured muscle or burned skin and bacterial endotoxins. Although many of these candidates will produce 'shock-like' states when given in large doses, they do not do so after doses that are likely to be released or produced by trauma.

Myocardial depressant factor has attracted considerable interest. It is a low molecular weight peptide or glycopeptide produced in the ischaemic pancreas. The myocardial depressant activity refers to its action in an isolated heart muscle preparation and not necessarily to its activity *in vivo*. Hence, its significance in 'shock' is not clear. Endogenous opioids may also have a 'toxic' depressant action on the cardiovascular system. The opioid antagonist naxalone raises blood pressure and improves survival after some forms of injury. It also raises blood pressure in patients with septic complications following surgery, however, this effect of naloxone is only transient and survival is not improved.

In conclusion, it seems unlikely that toxic factors initiate the general response to injury but they may subsequently be important in determining the outcome.

12.3.3 Afferent nervous impulses and CNS function

At the end of the last century, Crile concluded that 'surgical shock was due to an impairment or breakdown of the central vasomotor mechanism due to excessive nociceptive afferent stimuli'. It has since been demonstrated that the ability to withstand haemorrhage is impaired by simultaneous nociceptive stimuli which travel from the injured tissue to the brain along the spinothalamic tracts of the spinal cord. Once in the brain these afferents seem to have many targets, including the hindbrain, hypothalamus, and even the sensory cortex (Fig. 12.1).

If injury has been anticipated, the defence reaction will have been triggered. This reaction can be mimicked by electrical stimulation at a number of sites in the brain including the hypothalamus and the periaqueductal grey (PAG). Of these areas only the PAG appears capable of fully integrating the defence reaction. This reaction or preparation for flight or fight, involves excitation of the sympathetic nervous system in order to increase blood pressure and cardiac output and redistribute blood from areas such as skin and the splanchnic area to the skeletal muscles, where the blood vessels are dilated by sympathetic cholinergic fibres. It is important to emphasize that there is an increase in both blood pressure and heart rate; the normal baroreceptor-mediated reflex bradycardia in response to a rise in blood pressure is inhibited during the defence or alerting reaction. A similar inhibition of the baroreflex can be elicited by nociceptive afferent stimuli which may well be generated by tissue injury. It is not surprising therefore, that such an inhibition has been noted immediately following accidental injury in man, a change that may persist for several weeks.

Although fluid loss from the circulation is the most important cause of the general response to injury, it is important to be aware of the fact that this response may be modified by changes in the functioning of the central nervous system and by the presence of toxic factors.

12.4 The general response to injury

12.4.1 Compensation of fluid loss

A loss of fluid from the circulation reduces the venous return of blood to the heart. This reduces cardiac output, which in turn leads to a fall in arterial blood pressure. This lowering of blood pressure is sensed by the high-pressure baroreceptors in the aortic arch and carotid sinuses. The number of afferent impulses from these stretch receptors decreases and so their inhibitory influence on automatic sympathetic outflow from the

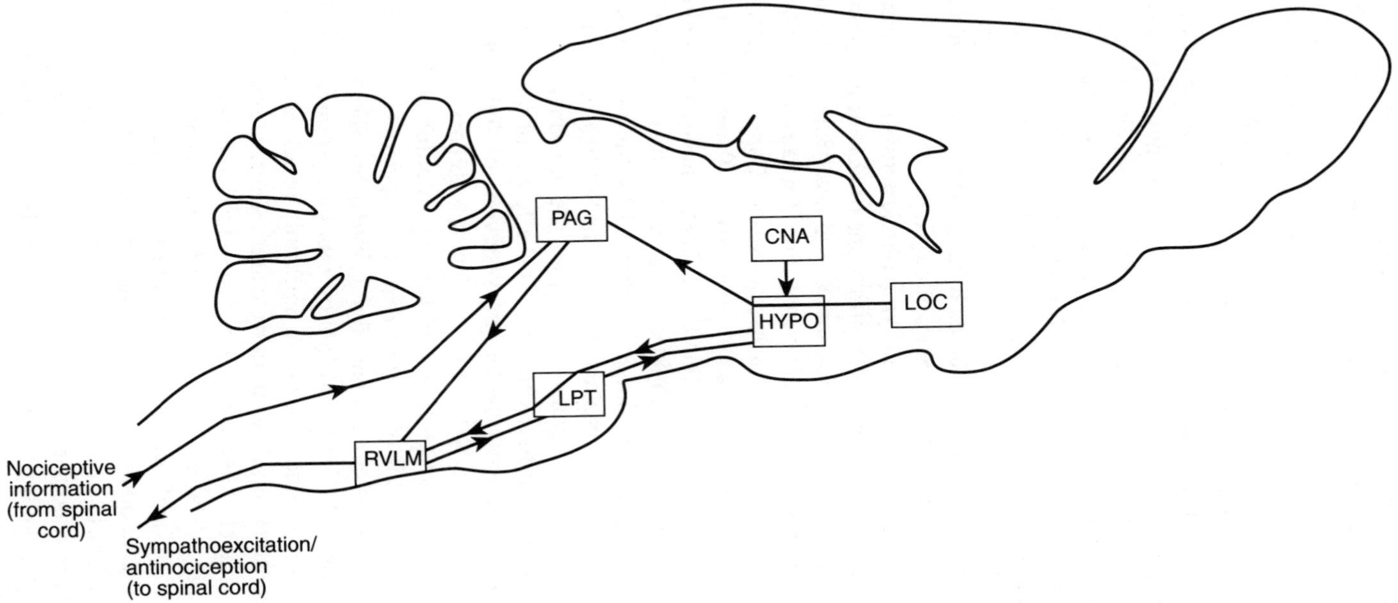

Fig. 12.1. Schematic diagram illustrating central nervous pathways which are involved in the visceral alerting response of the defence reaction and which may be involved in the cardiovascular and antinociceptive response to injury: CNA, central nucleus of the amygdala; HYPO, hypothalamus; LPT, lateral pontine tegmentum; LOC, lateral to the optic chiasma; PAG, periaqueductal grey; RVLM, rostral ventrolateral medulla.

central nervous system is reduced. Hence, a fall in blood pressure elicits a reflex increase in the activity of the sympathetic nervous system and a concomitant reduction in cardiac parasympathetic (vagal) activity (Fig. 12.2). The precise mechanisms involved are exceedingly complex but it seems that the baroreceptor afferents terminate in the nucleus tractus solitarius of the medulla. There is then a diffuse pattern of interconnections within the brainstem, finally converging on the autonomic pre-ganglionic neurones.

The increase in sympathetic activity is enhanced by stimulation of the peripheral chemoreceptors in the carotid and aortic bodies. The chemoreceptors are sensitive to hypoxia, which can be caused either by a reduction in arterial oxygen tension or by a local reduction in blood flow to the chemoreceptors. In addition, increases in carbon dioxide tension and falls in arterial blood pH increase the sensitivity of the arterial chemoreceptors to low oxygen levels. There are also central chemoreceptors, on the ventral surface of the medulla, which are stimulated by a rise in the carbon dioxide tension (and, hence, falls in pH) of cerebrospinal fluid.

What is the purpose of this increase in sympathetic activity? It increases the rate and strength of cardiac muscle contractions (that is, it has positive chronotropic and inotropic effects). The increase in heart rate will be augmented by the concomitant reduction in vagal tone. By causing peripheral vasoconstriction it also reduces the intravascular space. Constriction of the veins (capacitance vessels) is most important as some 70 per cent of the blood volume is normally contained within them. There will also be arteriolar constriction, which increases pre-capillary resistance, thereby lowering capillary hydrostatic pressure (the latter determined by the ratio between pre-capillary and post-capillary resistance). From the Starling equation (see p. 267) it can be seen that this change will favour the movement of tissue fluid into the circulation ('autotransfusion'). This effect is of most importance in skeletal muscle, which is the largest 'reservoir' of fluid for autotransfusion (Fig. 12.3). In a 70 kg man, a fall in capillary hydrostatic pressure of only 4–5 mmHg (0.6 kPa) can lead to an autotransfusion of 200–400 ml within 30 min. It is of interest that those species that are most resistant to haemorrhage (for example, flying birds) are those that can compensate most efficiently for blood loss by rapid autotransfusion. The increased vasoconstriction does not occur uniformly in all vascular beds; the coronary and cerebral vessels seem to be spared. Thus, in response to a reduction in circulating blood volume, there is a reduction in the size of the vascular bed that has to be perfused, the heart pumps more efficiently, tissue fluid is mobilized, and circulation is maintained to vital areas such as heart and brain. If the blood loss cannot be compensated and venous return continues to fall, the heart, under strong sympathetic drive, contracts vigorously. But because the chambers are not full, ventricular distortion receptors may be activated and provoke a striking reflex vagal bradycardia (Bezold–Jarisch reflex).

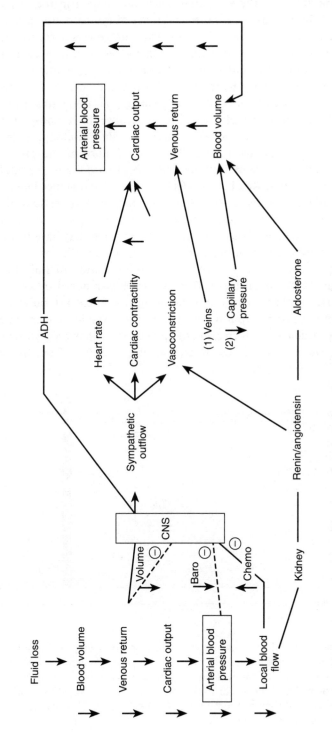

Fig. 12.2. Overview of a reflex compensation of fluid loss from the circulation.

The importance of the sympathetic nervous system in the response to injury is emphasized by the lowered resistance of sympathectomized animals to injury and the poor record of sympathetic antagonists in the treatment of shock. Unfortunately, vasoconstriction in tissues such as skeletal muscle cannot be maintained indefinitely. Sympathetic stimulation eventually causes a rise in capillary hydrostatic pressure and, hence, fluid tends to move out of the circulation. (This may be analogous to the state of irreversible or decompensated shock.) This occurs because the response of the pre-capillary resistance vessels to vasoconstrictor fibre discharge fails before that of the post-capillary vessels. This early failure of the pre-capillary response seems to be caused by the build-up of vasodilator metabolites in the ischaemic tissues. Red blood cells tend to sludge together late in shock and this will tend to raise post- rather than pre-capillary resistance.

Steroid treatment has frequently been advocated in shock. Although this treatment has no sound basis, one beneficial action it may have is the maintenance of vascular responsiveness to sympathetic stimulation.

Other mechanisms are involved in the compensation of fluid loss after injury (Fig. 12.2). Renal blood flow is markedly reduced by sympathetic vasoconstrictor fibre activity and the drop in afferent arteriolar pressure leads to an increased output of renin from the juxtaglomerular apparatus. This in turn leads to the formation of angiotensin, a powerful vasoconstrictor agent, which, through the liberation of aldosterone from the adrenal

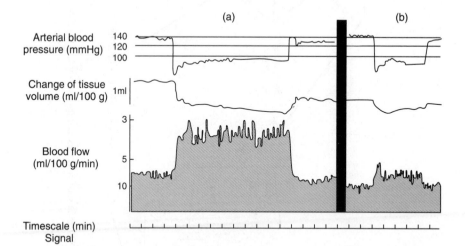

Fig. 12.3. Effect of haemorrhage on blood pressure, hind-quarter volume and blood flow in the chloralose-anaesthetised cat (a) before and (b) after cutting the regional sympathetic vasoconstrictor fibres. Note the progressive reduction in tissue volume in the innervated but not in the denervated tissues. From Oberg, B. (1964). *Acta Physiologica Scandinavica, Suppl.* 229.

cortex, enhances tubular sodium retention and, hence, fluid retention. Fluid conservation is also aided by an increase in the secretion of antidiuretic hormone (ADH) from the posterior lobe of the pituitary gland. One factor influencing the liberation of ADH is stimulation of receptors at the junction between the left atrium and the pulmonary veins (the low-pressure baroreceptors or 'volume' receptors). The injured patient commonly complains of thirst, probably mediated through the 'thirst centres' in the hypothalamus and will drink avidly. All the mechanisms described above will help to restore the intravascular volume. Deficits in erythrocytes and plasma protein concentrations require more long-term correction.

12.4.2 Neuroendocrine responses to injury

12.4.2.1 *Anterior pituitary gland*

The best known of the endocrine responses to injury are those involving the pituitary gland (Fig. 12.4). The secretion of adrenocorticotrophic hormone (ACTH) from the anterior pituitary (adenohypophysis) is controlled by corticotrophin-releasing hormone (CRH) from the hypothalamus; CRH is carried to the pituitary by the pituitary portal vessels. The secretion of CRH is enhanced by injury. This effect seems to be due to afferent stimuli travelling in the spinothalamic tract to the pons and, thence, via the medial

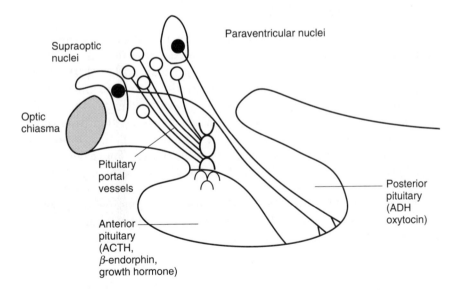

Fig. 12.4. Diagrammatic representation of neurosecretory cells in the hypothalamus showing how the axons of those in the supraoptic and paraventricular nuclei descend to the posterior pituitary where the axons of those that secrete hypothalamic-releasing hormones terminate about the vessels of the pituitary portal tract.

forebrain bundle, to the hypothalamus. The neurotransmitters involved in the control of CRH secretion are not all known, although secretion is stimulated by acetylcholine and inhibited by both noradrenalin and adrenalin.

As well as being involved in stimulation of the ACTH–adrenal cortex axis, CRH may also contribute to a number of the other responses to injury. For example, it stimulates efferent sympathetic activity, increases heat production, inhibits the baroreflex (see above), and modifies gastrointestinal function (reduces gastric emptying and small bowel transit and increases large bowel transit).

The arterial baroreceptors may provide another link between trauma and ACTH secretion. Stimulation of the baroreceptors inhibits ACTH secretion; this may be due to a direct noradrenergic projection from the nucleus tractus solitarius to the hypothalamus.

When ACTH is released from the anterior pituitary, it is accompanied by β-endorphin. As already mentioned, the endogenous opioids have been implicated in the development of 'shock' and it is suggested that pituitary endorphins act upon opioid receptors in the brain to depress cardiovascular function.

The secretion of prolactin and growth hormone (GH) is increased in humans after injury, however, the secretion of insulin-like growth factor which is responsible for many of the anabolic effects of GH is reduced.

12.4.2.2 *Posterior pituitary gland*

The neurones that synthesize ADH and oxytocin and secrete them in the posterior lobe of the pituitary (neurohypophysis) have their cell bodies in the magnocellular supraoptic and paraventricular nuclei of the hypothalamus. Both ADH and oxytocin are secreted in response to injury but the proportions in which they are secreted vary with different stimuli. The secretion of ADH is normally brought about by stimulation from osmoreceptors and, particularly after fluid loss from the circulation, by afferent vagal fibres from the 'volume' receptors in the thorax. The magnocellular nuclei are stimulated by cholinergic fibres and inhibited by noradrenergic ones.

The ability of ADH to raise blood pressure and conserve water are of obvious value after injury. This hormone may also play a role in injury-related metabolic changes such as the conversion of hepatic glycogen to glucose.

12.4.2.3 *Adrenal gland*

The sympathetic activation that occurs after injury increases secretion of catecholamines from the adrenal medulla. Although both adrenalin and noradrenalin are secreted in response to injury, adrenalin is the principal hormone in the adult. A particularly potent stimulus for secretion is a reduction in blood volume.

As far as the adrenal cortex is concerned, injury stimulates the hypothalamic–hypophyseal system to release ACTH, as outlined earlier, which in turn stimulates the secretion of corticosteroids from the cortex. Although this adrenocortical response to injury is well documented, its function is still not clear. Removal of the adrenal gland (adrenalectomy) greatly reduces resistance to injury. However, adrenalectomized animals maintained on constant doses of cortical hormones show a normal metabolic response to injury. This finding suggests that an increase in the secretion of corticosteroids is not necessary for expression of the metabolic responses to injury and has led to the concept that steroids play a 'permissive' role in shock. Raised concentrations of adrenocortical hormones are, however, necessary for the compensation of post-traumatic fluid loss. Aldosterone is also secreted from the adrenal cortex and, as already mentioned, promotes sodium retention in the kidney after injury.

12.4.2.4 *Pancreatic islets*

Injury affects the secretion of both insulin and glucagon from the pancreas. The secretion of these hormones is largely controlled by the plasma glucose concentration. However, it can be modified by the autonomic nervous system. Both stimulation of the sympathetic innervation of the pancreas and an increase in circulating adrenalin enhance glucagon secretion but decrease that of insulin. Parasympathetic stimulation increases insulin and glucagon secretion. Thus, after a mild injury, the plasma insulin concentration may be appropriate for the increased plasma glucose concentration but after more severe injuries, when glucose concentrations are even higher (see below), insulin concentrations may be lower than predicted because of intense sympathetic activation.

12.4.3 **The metabolic response to injury**

12.4.3.1 *Phases of the response*

The first phase of the metabolic response to injury begins with the mobilization of the body fuels. In fact mobilization may start before injury as part of the fight or flight response discussed earlier. This phase leads into the 'ebb' phase that immediately follows injury and is classically associated with an inhibition of thermoregulation at a time when oxygen transport is adequate. Most of the physiological responses already discussed in this chapter occur during this early 'ebb' phase. If the injury is overwhelming, the 'ebb' phase is followed by a phase of necrobiosis which precedes death. However, with recovery, the 'ebb' phase is followed by the 'flow' phase associated with an increase in metabolic activity.

12.4.3.2 *Mobilization of fuel stores*

The hydrolysis of tissue glycogen stores to raise extracellular glucose concentration and of triglycerides to form free fatty acids is largely due to sympathoadrenal medullary excitation and the release of hormones.

The principal glycogen stores are in liver and muscle (Fig. 12.5). However, these stores are very labile and the increased susceptibility to injury during starvation may be related to reduced glycogen stores. The hydrolysis of muscle glycogen after injury is largely due to the action of circulating catecholamines on β-adrenoceptors. The glycogen is hydrolysed to glucose-6-phosphate but not to glucose because glucose-6-phosphatase is absent from skeletal muscle. Instead glucose-6-phosphate is converted to pyruvate and lactate which pass into the circulation and are carried to the liver where they are converted to glucose (Cori cycle). The hydrolysis of liver glycogen can be caused by direct stimulation of the sympathetic innervation to the liver and, probably most importantly, by pancreatic glucagon. Antidiuretic hormone may also be an important factor in stimulating glycogenolysis after injury.

Lipid stores are mobilized after injury by direct activation of the sympathetic innervation to adipose tissue. The triacylglycerol (triglyceride) in adipose tissue is hydrolysed to form free or non-esterified fatty acids and glycerol. The free fatty acids are released into the circulation where they bind to albumin. The extent to which plasma free fatty acid concentration rises after injury will ultimately depend upon the blood flow through the

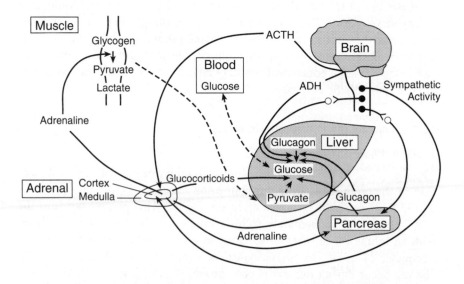

Fig. 12.5. Central nervous system stimulation of hepatic glucose output. From Frayn, K.N. (1977). *Metabolic responses to trauma.* Folio Traumatologia, Geigy, Basle.

adipose tissue and on the amount of albumin available to bind to the fatty acids. After major injuries and haemorrhage, blood flow in adipose tissue is markedly reduced and the concentration of free fatty acids in plasma does not rise as much as might be predicted from the level of sympathoadrenal activation.

12.4.3.3 *The 'ebb' phase*

At the time of injury the body's fuel stores may have been mobilized for fight or flight. Becuase it is not possible to replenish the fuel stores after injury, there is a need to conserve or husband any reserves that remain. This is what happens in the 'ebb' phase. For example, the utilization of glucose is inhibited in insulin-sensitive tissues.

In small mammals (for example, the rat), the 'ebb' phase is characterized by a fall in metabolic rate and body temperature. This is due to a central change in thermoregulation and not to a failure in oxygen delivery to thermogenic tissues. The inhibition of thermoregulation, which involves the central control of both heat production and heat loss, is a result of activating noradrenergic fibres supplying the hypothalamus. In humans there is no evidence for a fall in heat production during the 'ebb' phase and this may reflect the fact that humans, unlike rats, rely more on changes in heat loss than heat production for thermoregulation. Indeed, there is some clinical evidence for an inhibition of behavioural thermoregulation after injury. The injured patient selects a higher environmental temperature for comfort than would be predicted from their body temperature. The fall in body temperature seen after severe injuries in humans may be due to failure of oxygen transport rather than a central change in thermoregulation. However, when the temperature of severely injured people falls, they do not shiver as expected. This may be related to the fact that an adequate arterial baroreceptor input to the central nervous system is necessary for the maintenance of shivering.

The relative contribution of fat oxidation to total energy production is increased after injury. As a result the respiratory quotient quickly falls. (The respiratory quotient is the volume of CO_2 expired divided by the volume of O_2 consumed: a figure of 1.0 represents carbohydrate oxidation and 0.7 fat oxidation.) The conversion of fatty acids into ketone bodies in the liver is increased after injury. Ketone bodies (acetoacetate and β-hydroxybutyrate) can form an alternative fuel for skeletal muscle and brain although it is difficult to assess their quantitative importance.

Hyperglycaemia is a prominent feature of the 'ebb' phase. Although adrenergic activity is still high, the main reason for the hyperglycaemia is the reduction in glucose utilization in insulin-dependent tissues such as skeletal muscle. The impairment of glucose utilization is caused by a suppression of insulin secretion by the increased sympathetic activity (an

α-adrenoceptor effect on the insulin-secreting pancreatic β-cells) and to the development of resistance to insulin. This insulin resistance is mediated at least in part by the raised concentrations of growth hormone, adrenalin, and glucocorticoids, although the cytokines may also have a role. The removal of glucose from the blood will also be limited by the increased concentrations of free fatty acids and ketone bodies, whose utilization is limited only by supply (that is, as plasma concentration rises, tissue uptake also rises). The reduction in glucose utilization by the insulin-dependent tissues will spare this energy substrate for the brain (an insulin-independent organ), which uses largely glucose and, to a lesser extent, ketone bodies.

12.4.3.4 *Necrobiosis*

This is the phase of the metabolic response to injury that immediately precedes death. It is characterized by a failure of oxygen transport to the tissues. Whole-body oxygen consumption and body temperature continue to fall. Increasing hypoxia in the tissues increases anaerobic glucose utilization, which, with decreased gluconeogenesis, produces the low blood glucose and high blood lactate concentrations found terminally. A non-respiratory acidosis develops, with a fall in blood pH and in total buffering capacity of the body. The lactate:pyruvate and β-hydroxybutyrate:acetoacetate ratios rise in blood and tissues, indicating hypoxia in both the cytoplasm and the mitochondria.

12.4.3.5 *The 'flow' phase*

In the 'flow' or recovery phase, metabolic rate may be raised. The fracture of a long bone increases energy expenditure by something like 20 per cent; after a major burn, metabolic rate may be doubled. The increase in metabolic rate may be accompanied by increases in temperature, heart rate, and ventilation. This pattern of response has led to the term 'traumatic fever', which, it must be emphasized is not related to infection. The increase in metabolic rate is due to a number of factors which include, an upward resetting of metabolic activity, increased efferent sympathetic drive, increased substrate cycling, and the metabolic activity of the wound (an extra organ). The upward central resetting of metabolic activity involves both the cytokines and the prostaglandins.

During the 'flow' phase, the utilization of exogenous glucose remains impaired and fat is still the most important energy source. However, in order to provide the insulin-independent tissues, such as brain, with glucose, there is a breakdown of muscle protein. This supplies alanine and other amino acids, which are the main precursors for gluconeogenesis in the liver. This mobilization of gluconeogenic amino acids is facilitated by glucocorticoids.

Elevated plasma glucose concentrations normally inhibit the release of gluconeogenic precursors from skeletal muscle and, hence, limit hepatic gluconeogenesis. This control mechanism is lost in the injured patient. Thus, in the 'flow' phase, the rates of fat oxidation and glucose turnover can both be raised. It has been suggested that this pattern of response is mediated by high plasma glucagon concentrations and especially by the high glucagon:insulin ratio. The increased plasma concentrations of free fatty acids and ketone bodies may help to suppress or at least limit skeletal muscle protein breakdown and alanine release.

The loss of muscle protein after major injuries can be large and may even threaten life. This loss is reflected in an increased urinary excretion of nitrogen, mainly as urea, but also as creatine, creatinine, and 3-methylhistidine. The latter is formed by the methylation of histidine during its incorporation into myofibrillar protein. 3-Methylhistidine is then released when myofibrillar protein is degraded and, as it cannot be reutilized, is excreted unchanged. It can therefore be used as a quantitative marker of myofibrillar protein breakdown. The breakdown of lean body mass is also reflected in increased urinary losses of sulphate, phosphate, potassium, and zinc.

There is no doubt that patients lose weight after injury. The loss of lean body mass (predominantly muscle) is almost three times greater than the loss of fat. This loss of body protein is caused by a change in the balance between protein synthesis and protein breakdown. The picture is far from clear but it seems that there is a reduction in muscle protein synthesis after minor injuries or surgical operations, whereas, after more severe injuries, breakdown is also increased. The plasma proteins behave rather differently; some increase after injury whereas others decrease. Those that increase are the acute-phase reactants (for example, C-reactive protein and fibrinogen) produced in the liver. The cytokines (especially interleukin-6) are potent stimuli of acute-phase protein synthesis. The acute-phase reactants can be described as the plasma proteins which show an increase in concentration in the acute or early phase of inflammation. Plasma albumin concentration, on the other hand, decreases during the first week or so after injury. This is due both to a reduction in synthesis and to an increase in the movement of albumin into the extravascular space.

Further reading

Barton, R.N. (1987). The neuroendocrinology of physical injury. *Baillière's Clinical Endocrinology and Metabolism*, **1**, 355–74.

Barton, R.N., Frayn, K.N., and Little, R.A. (1990). Trauma, burns and surgery. In *The metabolic and molecular basis of acquired disease*, (ed. Cohen, R.D., Lewis, B., Alberti, K.G.M.M., and Denman, A.M.), pp. 684–717. Bailliere Tindall, London.

Fine, J. (1976). Shock and peripheral circulatory insufficiency. In *Handbook of physiology*, (ed. Hamilton, W.F.), Section 2, Circulation, Vol. III, pp. 2037–69.

Folkow, B. and Neil, E. (1971). *Circulation*. Oxford University Press, London.

Frayn, K.N. (1986). Hormonal control of metabolism in trauma and sepsis. *Clinical Endocrinology*, **24**, 577–99.

Little, R.A. and Kirkman, E. (1988). The pathophysiology of trauma and shock. In *Fluid resuscitation*, (ed. W. Kox, J. Gamble), pp. 467–82. Bailliere's Clinical Anaesthesiology, Vol. 2, No. 3.

Renkin, E.M. (1984). Control of microcirculation and blood–tissue exchange. In *Handbook of physiology*, Section 2, *The Cardiovascular System*, (ed. Renkin, E.M. and Michel, C.C.), Vol. IV—*Microcirculation*, part 2, pp. 627–87.

Wiggers, C.J. (1950). *Physiology of shock*. The Commonwealth Fund, New York.

INDEX